Effects of Physical Activity on Chronic Disease

Effects of Physical Activity on Chronic Disease

Editors

Yoshiaki Minakata
Kazuhisa Asai

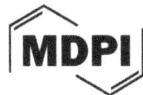

Basel • Beijing • Wuhan • Barcelona • Belgrade • Novi Sad • Cluj • Manchester

Editors
Yoshiaki Minakata
National Hospital
Organization Wakayama
Hospital
Wakayama
Japan

Kazuhisa Asai
Osaka Metropolitan
University
Osaka
Japan

Editorial Office
MDPI
St. Alban-Anlage 66
4052 Basel, Switzerland

This is a reprint of articles from the Special Issue published online in the open access journal *Journal of Clinical Medicine* (ISSN 2077-0383) (available at: https://www.mdpi.com/journal/jcm/special_issues/1ZJG867VE4).

For citation purposes, cite each article independently as indicated on the article page online and as indicated below:

Lastname, A.A.; Lastname, B.B. Article Title. *Journal Name* **Year**, *Volume Number*, Page Range.

ISBN 978-3-7258-0285-2 (Hbk)
ISBN 978-3-7258-0286-9 (PDF)
doi.org/10.3390/books978-3-7258-0286-9

© 2024 by the authors. Articles in this book are Open Access and distributed under the Creative Commons Attribution (CC BY) license. The book as a whole is distributed by MDPI under the terms and conditions of the Creative Commons Attribution-NonCommercial-NoDerivs (CC BY-NC-ND) license.

Contents

Hiroki Tashiro and Koichiro Takahashi
Clinical Impacts of Interventions for Physical Activity and Sedentary Behavior on Patients with Chronic Obstructive Pulmonary Disease
Reprinted from: *J. Clin. Med.* **2023**, *12*, 1631, doi:10.3390/jcm12041631 1

Yoshiaki Minakata, Yuichiro Azuma, Seigo Sasaki and Yusuke Murakami
Objective Measurement of Physical Activity and Sedentary Behavior in Patients with Chronic Obstructive Pulmonary Disease: Points to Keep in Mind during Evaluations
Reprinted from: *J. Clin. Med.* **2023**, *12*, 3254, doi:10.3390/jcm12093254 17

**Kentaro Ito, Maki Esumi, Seiya Esumi, Yuta Suzuki, Tadashi Sakaguchi,
Kentaro Fujiwara, et al.**
Physical Activity Estimated by the Wearable Device in Lung Disease Patients: Exploratory Analyses of Prospective Observational Study
Reprinted from: *J. Clin. Med.* **2023**, *12*, 4424, doi:10.3390/jcm12134424 32

**Yoshiki Nakahara, Shingo Mabu, Tsunahiko Hirano, Yoriyuki Murata, Keiko Doi,
Ayumi Fukatsu-Chikumoto and Kazuto Matsunaga**
Neural Network Approach to Investigating the Importance of Test Items for Predicting Physical Activity in Chronic Obstructive Pulmonary Disease
Reprinted from: *J. Clin. Med.* **2023**, *12*, 4297, doi:10.3390/jcm12134297 40

**Yoshikazu Yamaji, Tsunahiko Hirano, Hiromasa Ogawa, Ayumi Fukatsu-Chikumoto,
Kazuki Matsuda, Kazuki Hamada, et al.**
Utility of the Shortness of Breath in Daily Activities Questionnaire (SOBDA-Q) to Detect Sedentary Behavior in Patients with Chronic Obstructive Pulmonary Disease (COPD)
Reprinted from: *J. Clin. Med.* **2023**, *12*, 4105, doi:10.3390/jcm12124105 54

**Yoriyuki Murata, Tsunahiko Hirano, Keiko Doi, Ayumi Fukatsu-Chikumoto,
Kazuki Hamada, Keiji Oishi, et al.**
Computed Tomography Lung Density Analysis: An Imaging Biomarker Predicting Physical Inactivity in Chronic Obstructive Pulmonary Disease: A Pilot Study
Reprinted from: *J. Clin. Med.* **2023**, *12*, 2959, doi:10.3390/jcm12082959 65

**Yuichiro Azuma, Yoshiaki Minakata, Mai Kato, Masanori Tanaka, Yusuke Murakami,
Seigo Sasaki, et al.**
Validation of Simple Prediction Equations for Step Count in Japanese Patients with Chronic Obstructive Pulmonary Disease
Reprinted from: *J. Clin. Med.* **2022**, *11*, 5535, doi:10.3390/jcm11195535 76

**Yulieth Rivas-Campo, Agustín Aibar-Almazán, Carlos Rodríguez-López,
Diego Fernando Afanador-Restrepo, Patricia Alexandra García-Garro,
Yolanda Castellote-Caballero, et al.**
Enhancing Cognition in Older Adults with Mild Cognitive Impairment through High-Intensity Functional Training: A Single-Blind Randomized Controlled Trial
Reprinted from: *J. Clin. Med.* **2023**, *12*, 4049, doi:10.3390/jcm12124049 85

**Antonella Bianco, Francesco Russo, Isabella Franco, Giuseppe Riezzo, Rossella Donghia,
Ritanna Curci, et al.**
Enhanced Physical Capacity and Gastrointestinal Symptom Improvement in Southern Italian IBS Patients following Three Months of Moderate Aerobic Exercise
Reprinted from: *J. Clin. Med.* **2023**, *12*, 6786, doi:10.3390/jcm12216786 97

Bartłomiej Ptaszek, Szymon Podsiadło, Olga Czerwińska-Ledwig, Bartosz Zając,
Rafał Niżankowski, Piotr Mika and Aneta Teległów
The Influence of Interval Training Combined with Occlusion and Cooling on Selected Indicators of Blood, Muscle Metabolism and Oxidative Stress
Reprinted from: *J. Clin. Med.* **2023**, *12*, 7636, doi:10.3390/jcm12247636 . . . . **110**

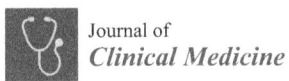

Review

Clinical Impacts of Interventions for Physical Activity and Sedentary Behavior on Patients with Chronic Obstructive Pulmonary Disease

Hiroki Tashiro and Koichiro Takahashi *

Division of Hematology, Respiratory Medicine and Oncology, Department of Internal Medicine, Faculty of Medicine, Saga University, Saga 849-8501, Japan
* Correspondence: takahak@cc.saga-u.ac.jp

Abstract: Recently, physical activity has increasingly become the focus in patients with chronic obstructive airway disease (COPD) because it is a strong predictor of COPD-related mortality. In addition, sedentary behavior, which is included as a category of physical inactivity including such behaviors as sitting or lying down, has an independent clinical impact on COPD patients. The present review examines clinical data related to physical activity, focusing on the definition, associated factors, beneficial effects, and biological mechanisms in patients with COPD and with respect to human health regardless of COPD. The data related to how sedentary behavior is associated with human health and COPD outcomes are also examined. Lastly, possible interventions to improve physical activity or sedentary behavior, such as bronchodilators and pulmonary rehabilitation with behavior modification, to ameliorate the pathophysiology of COPD patients are described. A better understanding of the clinical impact of physical activity or sedentary behavior may lead to the planning of a future intervention study to establish high-level evidence.

Keywords: chronic obstructive pulmonary disease; physical activity; sedentary behavior

1. Introduction

Chronic obstructive pulmonary disease (COPD) is a common respiratory disease, with 251 million cases worldwide, and it is a life-threatening disease that became the third leading cause of death globally in 2019 [1]. Medical interventions focusing on physical activity in the stable phase are currently demanded for COPD patients according to the results of several studies, although avoiding events such as exacerbations, infections, and comorbidities is also important because they are involved in clinical outcomes, including mortality, of COPD patients [2]. In addition, the specific impact of sedentary behavior on COPD patients has come to be understood [3]. Importantly, the effects of physical inactivity and sedentary behavior on clinical outcomes of COPD patients are different, and many data have shown that sedentary behavior negatively affects the pathophysiology of COPD, independent of physical inactivity, as described below.

In this review, the clinical impacts of physical activity and sedentary behavior on patients with COPD are addressed. The interactions of physical activity, sedentary behavior, and human health regardless of COPD are also described to explore novel therapeutic approaches. Lastly, possible therapeutic interventions focusing on sedentary behavior for COPD patients, including pharmacological and nonpharmacological interventions, such as pulmonary rehabilitation including behavior modification, are shown. We believe that the present review can contribute practically to clinical practice and provide future direction for the appropriate design of a clinical trial specifically focusing on sedentary behavior in COPD patients.

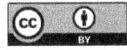

2. Physical Activity and Human Health

2.1. What Is Physical Activity?

Physical activity is defined as any movement or exercise of the body produced by skeletal muscles that requires energy consumption [4]. To focus on the clinical impact of physical activity on human health, the intensity level should be considered with respect to individual physical performance and response. Physical activity involves organs and tissues producing motion such as the skeletal muscles, heart, lungs, and others, and it leads to energy metabolism via aerobic or anaerobic pathways, depending on the individual threshold [5]. Aerobic metabolism requires oxygen to meet the energy demand during movement and uses energy derived from adenosine triphosphate (ATP) synthesized in the mitochondria of skeletal muscle by the tricarboxylic acid cycle [6,7]. Movements inducing aerobic metabolism are normally considered light- to moderate-intensity activities that allow people to perform typically repeating sequences of movements without causing risk or harm to human health [8,9]. On the other hand, anaerobic metabolism induces glycolysis, which is the transformation of glucose to lactate via the pyruvate cascade and synthesis of ATP under limited amounts of oxygen [10,11]. Movements inducing anaerobic metabolism are high-intensity activities that reach in excess of 90% of the maximum heart rate, increasing the risk of physical disorders such as musculoskeletal injuries along with the higher load on the body [12,13]. Thus, the recommended intensity level of an activity and its duration in daily life should be considered according to its benefit, especially for elderly individuals.

For standardized evaluation of physical activity, several methods including questionnaires and devices are used [14]. Briefly, questionnaires involve individual reporting of patients' own physical activity behaviors, along with job categories, such as the global physical activity questionnaire, international physical activity questionnaire, and the short physical performance battery [14,15]. Devices such as pedometers that count steps and accelerometers that measure truncal or limb movements are normally used [14]. Physical activity considering intensity and duration has increasingly come into focus for the maintenance of human health and the improvement of disease pathophysiology. The intensity of physical activity is calculated by metabolic equivalents (METs) and defined as follows: sedentary behavior, 1.0–1.5 METs; light intensity, less than 3.0 METs; moderate intensity, 3.0–6.0 METs; vigorous intensity, more than 6.0 METs [16]. Examples of physical activities calculated by METs are shown in Table 1.

Table 1. Examples of physical activities calculated by metabolic equivalents.

Major Headings of Physical Activity	METs
Sitting	1.5
Walking slowly	2
Standing performing light work	2–2.5
Walking at 3 mph	3.3
Walking at 4 mph	5
Walking at 4.5 mph	6.3
Jogging at 5 mph	8
Jogging at 6 mph	10
Running at 7 mph	11.5
Leisure Activities and Sports	
Arts, crafts, playing cards	1.5
Fishing, darts	2.5
Sailing, wind surfing	3
Table tennis	4
Golf	4.3
Badminton, basketball, volleyball	4.5–8
Tennis	5–8

Table 1. Cont.

Major Headings of Physical Activity	METs
Bicycling (10–12 mph)	6
Bicycling (14–10 mph)	10
Swimming—leisurely	6
Swimming—moderate/hard	8–11

METs: metabolic equivalents, mph: miles per hour. Data are cited from a paper by Haskell et al. [17].

The recommended intensity of physical activity differs depending on life stage, purpose, and demand. For example, it is strongly recommended that children and adolescents do at least an average of 60 min per day of moderate- to vigorous-intensity physical activity [18–20]. For adults aged 18–64 years, 150–300 min of moderate-intensity aerobic physical activity throughout the week and muscle-strengthening activity at moderate or greater intensity involving all major muscles groups on two or more days a week is strongly recommended [21,22]. For older adults aged 65 years and older, at least 150–300 min of moderate-intensity aerobic physical activity or 75–150 min of vigorous-intensity aerobic physical activity throughout the week is recommended [21,23]. Muscle-strengthening activities such as exercise training at moderate or greater intensity can also be performed on two or more days a week, along with the physical activity protocol mentioned above [4]. At all ages, physical activity should be undertaken as part of recreation, leisure such as play, games, sports, or planned exercise, transportation, work, or household chores in daily occupational, educational, home, and community settings [4], but the appropriate intensity level of the activity should be considered depending on the physical condition, including COPD and comorbidities. According to these recommendations, physical activity should be encouraged for maintenance of human health, although it is necessary to avoid excessive load on skeletal muscles that could cause harm.

2.2. Factors Associated with Physical Activity

Considering the clinical impact of physical activity on human health, it is necessary to understand which factors are related to physical activity in daily life. The factors associated with physical activity are varied, and include physical disability, mental health, lifestyle, and environmental situation. Physical function, including bone mass and muscle strength, tends to decrease with increasing age, which is related to decreased physical activity [23–25]. Specifically, sarcopenia, which is an age-related decrease of skeletal muscle volume plus low muscle strength, is associated with decreased physical performance [26]. Osteopenia/osteoporosis, which is characterized by low bone mass, also increases the risk of fractures due to bone fragility, leading to decreased physical activity [27,28]. The range of motion of the ankle joint, which is important for smooth forward movement during walking, is restricted by trauma, aging, and inflammatory disease of the joint [29,30] and, importantly, limited joint mobility decreases physical activity [30]. Mental health also contributes to physical inactivity [31]. Cross-sectional analyses involving 1536 Germans showed that individuals who do not perform physical exercise have a 3.15 times increased risk of developing moderate to severe depression [32]. Furthermore, positive mood, emotions [33,34], and even sleep quality are significantly correlated with physical activity level [35]. Lifestyles of individuals [36], including use of cell phones and computers, as well as playing video games, are also related to reductions in steps per day, and these data remind us of the necessity of 'behavior modification' to improve physical activity. Certainly, a person's environmental situation is a strong factor related to physical activity. Accordingly, various factors affect physical activity, and interventions for improvement require a multilateral focus.

2.3. Beneficial Effects of Physical Activity on Human Health and the Mechanisms

Improvement of physical activity produces beneficial effects on human health and quality of life (QOL) [4]. Evidence has shown that regular physical activity such as mat

Pilates improves physical function, including muscle strength, flexibility, and cardiorespiratory fitness [37]. Importantly, physical activity increases life expectancy [38]. A multicenter, cohort analysis in the US showed that a greater number of daily steps measured by accelerometer is significantly associated with lower all-cause mortality [39]. Notably, whether an intervention that increases physical activity would contribute to increasing life expectancy is not known because of the lack of clinical studies, but all-cause mortality might be reduced by improving wellbeing with increased individual physical activity. Furthermore, physical activity can contribute to health benefits for adults and older adults with chronic conditions, such as cancer survivors, or those with hypertension or type 2 diabetes mellitus. Briefly, a higher intensity of physical activity after cancer diagnosis has a protective effect on all-cause and cancer-specific mortality of various types of cancer [40]. For hypertension, people who engage in regular exercise show decreased systolic blood pressure of approximately 12 mmHg compared to people who do not exercise regularly [41]. Aerobic activity and/or muscle-strengthening activity are also related to improvements in glucose tolerance assessed as by glycosylated hemoglobin and insulin levels in patients with type 2 diabetes mellitus [42]. In terms of mental health, several studies have shown that engaging in physical activity and/or exercise programs can also improve emotional wellbeing [43]. Babyak et al. reported that an aerobic exercise intervention showed significantly better improvement and a lower relapse rate of depression than psychotropic treatment [44]. Similarly, a walking program in addition to social sports, measured using a 10-item modified version of the social support for exercise scale [45], was significantly associated with greater positive mood in women [46]. Notably, exercise, as mentioned above, is defined as planned, structured, and repetitive physical activity, not exactly identical to the broad meaning of physical activity [47]. However, exercise training has the capacity to improve physical activity with modification of behavior [47].

As for the biological mechanisms of the beneficial effects of improvement of physical activity, blunting or optimizing modulation of hormonal stress-responsive systems such as the hypothalamic–pituitary–adrenal axis and the sympathetic nervous system, which contribute to physiological, emotional, and metabolic reactivity, has been considered [48–51]. In addition, exercise affects the brain by enhancing growth factor expression and neural plasticity, contributing to improved mood and cognition [52,53]. A resilient anti-inflammatory effect through minimization of excessive inflammation is also induced by regular exercise/activity, which is supported by previous studies. Briefly, cancers, hypertension, and type 2 diabetes mellitus are associated with systemic markers of inflammation such as tumor necrosis factor-alpha, interleukin (IL)-1, IL-6, IL-8, and C-reactive protein, and exercise intervention reduces them [48]. As mentioned above, exercise intervention increases physical activity along with improvements of skeletal muscle function and cardiopulmonary function, and the improvement might attenuate systemic inflammation [54,55]. According to these data, exploring biological targets related to improvement of physical activity might be important for focusing on novel therapeutic perspectives.

3. Physical Activity and Chronic Obstructive Pulmonary Disease

3.1. Clinical Impact of Physical Activity in Patients with COPD

There is increasing evidence that decreased physical activity in patients with COPD is an important part of the pathophysiology that is associated with the clinical outcome. For example, Minakata et al. [56] reported that patients with COPD showed a significant reduction in the duration of physical activity, including activities at each intensity level of more than 2.0 METs, 2.5 METs, 3.0 METs, and 3.5 METs, compared to healthy subjects. In addition, levels of physical activity were further reduced with progression of the Global Initiative for Chronic Obstructive Lung Disease (GOLD) stage [56]. Similarly, walking and standing times are shorter, and time spent sitting and lying down is longer in patients with COPD than in healthy subjects [57]. Another single-center study showed that, in patients with COPD, daily physical activity measured by a triaxial accelerometer was an independent prognostic factor for mortality and hospitalization due to severe exacerbations [58]. Importantly, Waschki et al. [59] suggested, in a prospective, cohort study, that physical activity is the most important predictor of all-cause mortality. The relative risks of death with a standardized decrease in physical activity level measured by a multisensory armband and steps per day are higher than those with worsening of pulmonary function, exercise capacity assessed by 6 min walk distance, COPD-related QOL, or symptoms such as dyspnea in patients with COPD.

Notably, sarcopenia [60], osteopenia [61], and depression [62] are negatively associated with physical activity, as mentioned above, and they are major comorbidities of COPD. Thus, a decreased level of physical activity in patients with COPD might be involved in these comorbidities. According to these data, physical activity has a great impact in patients with COPD, and aggressive intervention to increase physical activity might be necessary to improve clinical outcomes of patients with COPD. Therefore, the present GOLD guideline notes that physical activity is a strong predictor of mortality, and COPD patients might be encouraged to increase their physical activity levels [63]. Again, it is unknown whether interventions that increase physical activity in patients with COPD, such as pulmonary rehabilitation, would directly contribute to improvement in the clinical outcomes of COPD, such as mortality, QOL, symptoms, and exacerbations, because of a shortage of data. Recently, a standard for the recommended number of steps for patients with COPD considering the modified Medical Research Council (mMRC) dyspnea scale and inspiratory capacity (IC) has been reported. A simple standard equation is the following: step count = $(-0.079 \times [age] - 1.595 \times [mMRC] + 2.078 \times [IC] + 18.149)^3$ [64], which is a useful tool for education of patients with COPD.

3.2. Factors Associated with Physical Activity in Patients with COPD

There are several factors related to physical activity in patients with COPD. Pulmonary function parameters such as forced vital capacity (FVC) percent predicted and FEV1.0 percent predicted are positively correlated with physical activity [56]. Results on the incremental shuttle walk test and 6 min walking distance, muscle function measured by handgrip force and quadriceps force, and symptoms such as dyspnea are also associated with physical activity in patients with COPD [57,65]. Briefly, skeletal muscle is positively associated with exercise capacity as assessed by 6 min walking distance and oxygen uptake at peak exercise measured by cardiopulmonary exercise testing in patients with COPD [66,67]. Interestingly, the cross-sectional area of skeletal muscle measured by computed tomography is positively associated with physical activity [67], showing that exercise capacity involves physical activities via skeletal muscle mass. Waschiki et al. [65] reported that physical activity measured by a multisensory armband and steps per day is negatively correlated with score on the modified Medical Research Council dyspnea scale. These data show that pulmonary function, exercise tolerance involving skeletal muscles, and symptoms related to COPD, which are major pathophysiological markers and clinical features of COPD, affect physical activity. Yoshida et al. reported that depression and anxiety assessed using the self-rating depression scale and state-trait anxiety inventory were significantly correlated with physical activity level [68]. Others also found, in a prospective, multicenter study, that symptoms of depression examined by the Hospital Anxiety and Depression Scale [69] were associated with a measurable reduction in physical activity 6 months later in patients with COPD [70]. In addition to parameters related to the pathophysiology of COPD, sociodemographic factors including age, sex, cultural group, educational level, and working status might be involved in physical activity levels [71]. Lifestyle and environmental factors including alcohol consumption and smoking might also be associated with physical activity levels in patients with COPD [71].

3.3. Possible Biomarkers Reflecting Physical Activity of Patients with COPD

There is an increased focus on evaluation of biomarkers related to physical activity in patients with COPD. For example, the total cholesterol level in blood, which reflects cardiac function and nutritional status, 8-isoprostane in exhaled breath condensate (EBC), which is an airway oxidative stress marker, and IL-6 in EBC, which reflects systemic inflammation, are negatively correlated with physical activity level [68,72]. Myokines, especially irisin, which has been discovered as a hormone secreted from skeletal myocytes at the start of exercise training [73,74], is considered a valuable biomarker reflecting physical activity in COPD. Ijiri et al. [75] evaluated serum irisin levels, where were lower in patients with COPD than in control subjects. The irisin level is correlated with physical activity level, but it is not correlated with pulmonary function and 6 min walking distance in patients with COPD. Interestingly, 8 week exercise training is linked to a significant increase in the irisin level [75], suggesting that irisin might be a useful candidate biomarker reflecting physical activity in patients with COPD. Furthermore, decreased serum irisin levels are involved in epithelial apoptosis, resulting in emphysema in patients with COPD [76]. Others have reported that growth differentiation factor 11 (GDF-11) in plasma, which is expressed in skeletal muscle and is linked to rejuvenating effects such as muscle regeneration, was positively correlated with physical activity level. GDF-11 is increased with improvements of lung function, quadriceps strength, and exercise capacity, as well as reduced inflammatory markers in patients with COPD [77]. According to these data, irisin and GDF-11 are beneficial, and 8-isoprostane has a harmful effect for COPD patients with respect to physical activity.

3.4. Beneficial Effects of Physical Activity on Patients with COPD and the Mechanisms

Previous epidemiological data have shown that increased physical activity is associated with the possible improvement of all-cause mortality or COPD-related mortality [58,59]. However, to the best of our knowledge, effects on mortality by specific physical activity interventions have not been evaluated. A multidisciplinary, exercise-based program aimed to improve physical activity such as pulmonary rehabilitation is considered a beneficial intervention [78–80], and pulmonary rehabilitation is strongly recommended in the present COPD guideline [81], because functional disorders of skeletal muscle, such as frailty or sarcopenia, have harmful impacts on the pathophysiology of COPD, including on physical activity [82,83]. There are several lines of evidence showing that pulmonary rehabilitation, physical activity programs including exercise in water, active mind-body movement therapies, neuromuscular electrical stimulation, and personalized physical activity programs with a motivational interview can reduce exacerbations and symptoms, including dyspnea and fatigue, as well as enhance health-related QOL, along with an improvement of physical activity in patients with COPD [84–87]. COPD-related QOL, symptoms including fatigue and dyspnea, and emotional function are also improved by pulmonary rehabilitation compared to usual care [86]. Notably, high-intensity exercise training with a 30 min exercise session at 80% of baseline maximal power output improves exercise capacity with physiological adaptation to endurance training occurring if the program is completed [88,89]. Importantly, it is still unclear whether pulmonary rehabilitation contributes to improvement of physical activity via exercise capacity, because physical activity is affected by several factors, such as sociodemographic factors, lifestyle, and environmental factors, along with individual exercise capacity, as mentioned above. Therefore, pulmonary rehabilitation might contribute to improvement in physical activity, potentially increasing physical function in patients with COPD, but further data are needed.

As an extrapulmonary comorbidity, depression is important in patients with COPD [62,90], and it involves physical activity, as mentioned above. Importantly, pulmonary rehabilitation also improves anxiety and depression as examined by the Hospital Anxiety and Depression Scale [91]. These data show that pulmonary rehabilitation might improve physical activity through a psychological effect, and improvement of anxiety and depression might also improve physical activity. Unfortunately, the biological mechanisms of the beneficial effects on physical activity for patients with COPD are still unclear because of the lack of clinical studies. Therefore, prospective interventional studies of physical activity in patients with COPD, especially those focusing on biological mechanisms such as hormonal stress-responsive systems, anti-inflammatory effects, and neural effects through the brain, should be performed.

4. Importance of Sedentary Behavior in Human Health

4.1. What Is Sedentary Behavior?

Sedentary behavior involves physically inactivity, with examples including sitting or lying down [92]. Sedentary behavior is more precisely defined as any waking behavior characterized by any energy expenditure less than or equal to 1.5 METs [16]. There is increasing evidence that sedentary behavior affects human health. The US National Health and Nutrition Examination Survey found that individuals, including children and adults, are generally sedentary for approximately 55% of their waking lives [93]. The degree to which sedentary behavior and physical activity interact in their association with health status is interesting. Biswas et al. [94] reported, in a meta-analysis, associations between physical activity and various deleterious health outcomes, and that sedentary time, independent of physical activity, is positively associated with all-cause mortality and cardiovascular disease-related mortality. Given the data, sedentary behavior, which might differ from a lack of moderate to vigorous physical activity, has qualitatively and independently harmful effects on health outcomes, human metabolism, and physical function. Katzmarzyk et al. [95] performed a prospective study to examine the relationship between sitting time and mortality in a representative sample of 17,013 Canadians ranging in age from 18 to 90 years. It was found that all-cause and cardiovascular disease-related mortalities were significantly higher if sitting time was increased, and the results remained significant after adjustment for potential confounders including physical activity level, which showed that sitting time had a harmful effect on mortality, independent of the physical activity level. Others reported that sedentary time measured by an accelerometer is associated with increases in waist circumference, triglycerides, 2 h plasma glucose, and insulin levels [96–98]. In addition, there is a relationship between sedentary behavior and reduced bone mass, and a 1% to 4% reduction was seen in the lumbar spine and femoral necks of healthy individuals following 12 weeks of bed rest [99].

Notably, sedentary behavior and physical inactivity do not have completely identical meanings, and careful interpretation of the studies mentioned above is needed, because physical inactivity constitutes an insufficient amount of moderate-to-vigorous physical activity [100], which is different from the definition of sedentary behavior, as mentioned above. In addition, a lifestyle in which time is spent performing an insufficient amount of moderate-to-vigorous physical activity does not directly involve increasing time spent being sedentary. Thus, sedentary behavior might have an impact on clinical outcomes independent of physical inactivity. According to these data, sedentary behavior is also an important independent factor along with general physical activity level, and shortening sedentary behavior time in daily life has beneficial effects on human health.

4.2. Factors Associated with Sedentary Behavior

Examples of sedentary behavior primarily consist of sitting and lying while watching TV, working on a computer, driving, eating, etc. There are many factors related to the duration of sedentary behavior, including sociodemographic phenotypes, such as age and sex. The amount of time spent on sedentary behavior is significantly greater with increased age in youths and adults, and it is also different between males and females in each age group among youths and adults aged 20–29, 60–69, and 70–85 years. Briefly, females spend more time sedentary than do males throughout youth and early adulthood, but this phenomenon is reversed after the age of 60 years [93]. Ethnic group is also associated with sedentary time, with Mexican Americans being less sedentary than their White counterparts in youth and adulthood [93]. Obesity, cancer, and chronic diseases including cardiovascular disease, hypertension, and diabetes mellitus, as well as psychosocial health, are also factors associated with sedentary behavior, even though whether they are the cause or the effect is unclear from the results of studies. Obesity can increase sedentary behavior because of structural and functional limitations to movement it can cause, and vice versa [101]. For children aged 7 to 11 years, TV watching and video game playing increase the risk of overweight by 17–44% and of obesity by 10–61% [102]. As for adults, Brown et al. [103]

analyzed 8071 middle-aged women, and participants who spent time sitting for more than 4.5 h per day were more likely to gain more than 5 kg than those who spent time sitting less than 3 h per day [104]. Increasing TV watching time or sitting at work for 2 h per day was also associated with an increased risk of obesity in adults. In terms of the relationship between cancer and sedentary behavior, a large, prospective, cohort study of 488,720 people aged 50 to 71 years showed that longer TV and video watching time was significantly associated with increased risks of colon cancer and endometrial cancer [105,106]. In chronic disease, sedentary time is positively associated with increased risks of cardiovascular disease [107], hypertension, [108] and diabetes mellitus [109].

In terms of psychosocial health, people with the highest level of sedentary behavior showed a 31% higher risk of mental disorders compared with less sedentary individuals [110], which indicated that psychosocial health might be an important factor associated with sedentary behavior, although strong evidence, such as from a prospective intervention study, is lacking. According to these data, various factors might be associated with sedentary behavior, but biological mechanisms for reducing sedentary behavior time to obtain a beneficial effect are unclear because of the absence of interventional studies.

5. Clinical Impact of Sedentary Behavior in Patients with Chronic Obstructive Pulmonary Disease

5.1. Clinical Impact of Sedentary Behavior in Patients with COPD

Evidence and studies show that sedentary behavior is associated with clinical outcomes in patients with COPD. Sedentary behavior including sitting and lying down during the day, as measured by triaxial accelerometers, accounts for a very high percentage, approximately 64%, of patients with COPD, higher than the 46% for healthy subjects, and both time spent sitting and time spent lying down are significantly longer in patients with COPD than in healthy subjects [57]. Another retrospective, cohort study showed that sedentary behavior was independently related to mortality in patients with COPD [3]. In this study involving 101 patients with COPD, time spent on sedentary behavior, defined as <1.5 METs as measured by activity monitors, was determined, and 41 patients died during the average follow-up period of 62 months. Sedentary behavior, especially more than 8.5 h per day spent in sedentary activities at <1.5 METs, was significantly correlated with mortality in patients with COPD after adjusting for potential confounders such as sex, age, body mass index, educational level, lung function, functional exercise capacity, and moderate-to-vigorous physical activity.

Interestingly, sedentary behavior itself might increase the risk of COPD. A large-scale, cross-sectional study of 14,073 individuals showed that those who remained sedentary for more than 7 h per day were more likely to have COPD than the control group, whose sedentary time was less than 3 h after adjustment for confounders including sex, age, country, educational level, marital status, occupation, economic status, smoking habit, physical activity, and all other chronic diseases, even though detailed physical activity levels other than sedentary time were not clarified [111]. Thus, increasing sedentary behavior time might contribute to increasing the incidence rate of COPD, along with the associated clinical outcomes.

5.2. Factors Possibly Associated with Sedentary Behavior in Patients with COPD

Evidence-based factors associated with sedentary behavior in patients with COPD are limited, but possible factors are considered to include COPD-related symptoms such as dyspnea and shortness of breath, reduced pulmonary function, weight loss including loss of skeletal muscle mass, decreased exercise capacity, and mental disorders such as depression. The pathophysiology of COPD involves airway narrowing as reflected by obstructive ventilatory failure on pulmonary function testing, which shows dyspnea and shortness of breath induced by dynamic pulmonary hyperinflation and oxygen desaturation [112]. Importantly, exercise can exacerbate the phenomena [113] that might contribute to avoidance of moderate or vigorous physical activity and increase sedentary behavior.

Even worse, the sequence of behavior induces a negative feedback cycle leading to poor outcomes for COPD patients, because increasing sedentary time with a reduction in physical activity contributes to skeletal muscle atrophy, especially in antigravity muscles such as the erector spinae muscles and thigh muscles, causing weight loss and decreased exercise capacity [59,66,67,114]. Consequently, the symptoms of dyspnea and shortness of breath are induced at a low intensity of physical activity, and patients try to avoid movement along with progression of muscle atrophy. Thus, interventions such as bronchodilators for symptom reduction and/or pulmonary rehabilitation with behavior modification are necessary to break these negative feedback cycles and improve COPD outcomes if we are to consider therapeutic intervention to improve physical activity and decrease sedentary behavior.

Mental disorders are also associated with sedentary behavior in patients with COPD. Indeed, anxiety and depression are important comorbidities in patients with COPD, and their prevalence was 80% in patients with COPD in a US cohort [90] and 38% in Japan [115]. As mentioned above, mental disorders are known to generally contribute to increased sedentary behavior [110], meaning they are also likely associated with sedentary behavior in patients with COPD. According to these data, various factors might be associated with sedentary behavior in patients with COPD, but biological mechanisms that can inform strategies for reducing sedentary behavior time and achieve a beneficial effect still remain unclear because of the shortage of interventional studies.

6. Possible Interventions Focused on Physical Activity, Especially Sedentary Behavior, in Patients with Chronic Obstructive Pulmonary Disease

6.1. Pharmacological Intervention: Bronchodilators

Use of bronchodilators is one of the pivotal treatment modalities for patients with COPD. Several interventional studies of bronchodilators showed their potential in improving sedentary behavior. Minakata et al. [116] performed a post hoc analysis of a randomized, double-blind, active-controlled, crossover trial (VESUTO study) that evaluated the efficacy of tiotropium plus olodaterol dual therapy versus tiotropium monotherapy in Japanese patients with COPD. Sedentary behavior was measured by a three-axis accelerometer, and 182 patients were evaluated to identify the impact of the bronchodilator treatments on sedentary behavior. It was found that sedentary behavior was significantly reduced by dual therapy, with an 8.64 min grater reduction in 1.0–1.5 METs of activity per day, compared to monotherapy, along with improvement of lung function and dyspnea.

In another study, we conducted a prospective, multicenter, randomized, open-label, parallel, interventional trial (SCOPE study) to examine the efficacy of tiotropium plus olodaterol dual therapy versus tiotropium monotherapy [117]. Importantly, the recruited patients with COPD in this study were treatment-naïve, which allowed us to effectively and specifically examine the impact of the treatments on sedentary behavior. Sedentary behavior, defined as activity of 1.0–1.5 METs measured by a triaxial accelerometer, was assessed, and 74 patients were enrolled. It was found that the duration of sedentary behavior after dual therapy tended to be reduced by more than 38.7 min per day compared to after monotherapy. Other parameters, such as changes of forced expiratory volume in 1 s and the transient dyspnea index, were more improved by dual therapy than monotherapy. We also reported that COPD patients with lower inspiratory capacity or shorter time spent on activity of more than 2.0 METs before dual therapy had a significantly greater reduction in sedentary time after dual therapy [118]. These data showed that sedentary behavior time was reduced because of improvement of decreased inspiratory capacity, which contributes to shortness of breath and dyspnea, by dual bronchodilator therapy. Recently, inhaled corticosteroid therapy was also found to be effective for patients with COPD, especially in those with frequent exacerbations with elevation of blood eosinophil levels [114,119]. We do not know the impact of inhaled corticosteroid therapy on sedentary behavior in patients with COPD, and further trials are needed to clarify its efficacy.

6.2. Nonpharmacological Intervention: Rehabilitation and Behavior Modification

Several interventional studies focusing on exercise rehabilitation and behavior modification showing beneficial outcomes related to sedentary behavior in patients with COPD have been reported. For example, Breyer et al. [120] reported that COPD patients were assigned to 2 h instruction by a professional Nordic walking instructor and performed a 3 month long training regimen. The training significantly reduced sitting time, and the improvement continued for 9 months after the intervention. Another trial showed that a home-based rehabilitation program and hospital-based rehabilitation program significantly reduced sedentary time and reduced acute exacerbations and emergency department visits in patients with COPD [121]. However, in a randomized, controlled trial, an intervention of ground-based walking training performed for between 30 and 45 min, two or three times a week for 8 to 10 weeks, showed no significant effect on sedentary time in patients with COPD [122]. According to these data, what constitutes effective and appropriate exercise rehabilitation to reduce sedentary time in patients with COPD is still unclear, and further interventional studies are needed.

Behavior modification might also be considered an effective intervention to improve physical activity and may be especially useful for reduction of sedentary behavior time. For example, Cruz et al. [123] reported a randomized, controlled trial in which COPD patients in the experimental group received a physical activity-focused behavioral intervention, which involved psychosocial support and education from physiotherapists, and use of a diary log to record daily steps during 3 months of pulmonary rehabilitation, with an additional 3 months of follow-up. Compared to the control group, the experimental group showed significantly reduced time of sedentary activities, along with increased moderate-to-vigorous physical activity. However, in another randomized, controlled trial performed by Cheng et al. [124], COPD patients performed a 6 week behavior change intervention that consisted of once weekly sessions for 6 weeks with a physiotherapist to reduce sedentary behavior through education, guided goal-setting, and real-time feedback. Compared to the sham intervention group, the intervention did not reduce sedentary behavior time. Considering these data, the clinical impact of exercise rehabilitation and behavior modification for sedentary behavior in patients with COPD remains controversial, and further trials are needed for clarification (Figure 1).

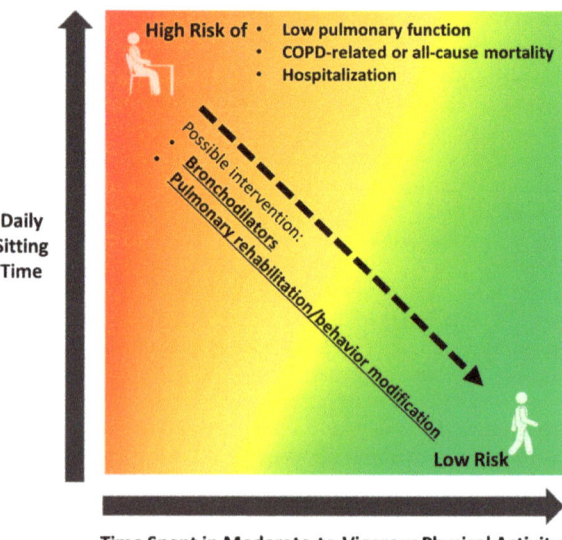

Figure 1. Risk of poor clinical outcomes of chronic obstructive pulmonary disease depending on physical activity and sedentary behavior, focusing on possible intervention.

The heat map shows that less sitting time and more moderate-to-vigorous physical activity are related to a reduced risk of poor clinical outcomes of chronic obstructive pulmonary disease. Interventions with bronchodilator therapy and pulmonary rehabilitation with behavior modification can possibly reduce the risk, which is indicated as decreasing from the red to the green. The figure is based on the reports from the 2018 Physical Activity Guidelines Advisory Committee Scientific Report [14], with partial modification.

7. Conclusions

The data reviewed above show the clinical impact of physical activity and sedentary behavior in patients with COPD, along with the benefit of physical activity for healthy individuals. Sedentary behavior affects clinical outcomes of COPD independent of physical inactivity, and interventions to reduce sedentary behavior time are necessary despite the difficulty presented by the multiplicity of related factors, including lifestyle and environmental factors, along with physical disorders. To break the negative feedback cycle of worsening clinical outcomes in patients with COPD induced by increasing sedentary behavior, bronchodilator and pulmonary rehabilitation with behavior modification appear to be effective for improvement of physical activity and sedentary behavior. Further investigations, such as those with a prospective design, large population, and multilateral focus including pharmacological and nonpharmacological approaches, are needed to obtain high-level evidence.

Author Contributions: H.T. and K.T. prepared the manuscript and checked the final manuscript. All authors have read and agreed to the published version of the manuscript.

Funding: This research did not receive any specific grant from funding agencies in the public, commercial, or not-for-profit sectors.

Institutional Review Board Statement: Not applicable.

Informed Consent Statement: Not applicable.

Data Availability Statement: Not applicable.

Conflicts of Interest: The authors declare no conflict of interest.

References

1. World Health Organization. Chronic Obstructive Pulmonary Disease (COPD). Available online: https://www.who.int/news-room/fact-sheets/detail/chronic-obstructive-pulmonary-disease-(copd).
2. Donaldson, G.C.; Seemungal, T.A.; Bhowmik, A.; Wedzicha, J.A. Relationship between exacerbation frequency and lung function decline in chronic obstructive pulmonary disease. *Thorax* **2002**, *57*, 847–852. [CrossRef] [PubMed]
3. Furlanetto, K.C.; Donária, L.; Schneider, L.P.; Lopes, J.R.; Ribeiro, M.; Fernandes, K.B.; A Hernandes, N.; Pitta, F. Sedentary Behavior Is an Independent Predictor of Mortality in Subjects With COPD. *Respir. Care* **2017**, *62*, 579–587. [CrossRef] [PubMed]
4. World Health Organization. *WHO Guidelines on Physical Activity and Sedentary Behaviour*; World Health Organization: Geneva, Switzerland, 2020; Available online: https://www.who.int/publications/i/item/9789240015128.
5. Hollmann, W.; Struder, H.K.; Tagarakis, C.V.; King, G. Physical activity and the elderly. *Eur. J. Prev. Cardiol.* **2007**, *14*, 730–739. [CrossRef] [PubMed]
6. Fernie, A.R.; Carrari, F.; Sweetlove, L.J. Respiratory metabolism: Glycolysis, the TCA cycle and mitochondrial electron transport. *Curr. Opin. Plant Biol.* **2004**, *7*, 254–261. [CrossRef]
7. Das, J. The role of mitochondrial respiration in physiological and evolutionary adaptation. *Bioessays* **2006**, *28*, 890–901. [CrossRef]
8. Best, J.R. Effects of Physical Activity on Children's Executive Function: Contributions of Experimental Research on Aerobic Exercise. *Dev. Rev.* **2010**, *30*, 331–551. [CrossRef]
9. Swain, D.P.; Franklin, B.A. Comparison of cardioprotective benefits of vigorous versus moderate intensity aerobic exercise. *Am. J. Cardiol.* **2006**, *97*, 141–147. [CrossRef]
10. Huckabee, W.E. Relationships of pyruvate and lactate during anaerobic metabolism. I. Effects of infusion of pyruvate or glucose and of hyperventilation. *J. Clin. Investig.* **1958**, *37*, 244–254. [CrossRef]
11. Huckabee, W.E. Relationships of pyruvate and lactate during anaerobic metabolism. II. Exercise and formation of O-debt. *J. Clin. Investig.* **1958**, *37*, 255–263. [CrossRef]
12. Ko, K.J.; Ha, G.C.; Kim, D.W.; Kang, S.J. Effects of lower extremity injuries on aerobic exercise capacity, anaerobic power, and knee isokinetic muscular function in high school soccer players. *J. Phys. Ther. Sci.* **2017**, *29*, 1715–1719. [CrossRef]
13. Jones, B.H.; Cowan, D.N.; Knapik, J.J. Exercise, training and injuries. *Sports Med.* **1994**, *18*, 202–214. [CrossRef] [PubMed]

14. 2018 Physical Activity Guidelines Advisory Committee. *2018 Physical Activity Guidelines Advisory Committee Scientific Report*; U.S. Department of Health and Human Services: Washington, DC, USA, 2018.
15. Guralnik, J.M.; Simonsick, E.M.; Ferrucci, L.; Glynn, R.J.; Berkman, L.F.; Blazer, D.G.; Scherr, P.A.; Wallace, R.B. A short physical performance battery assessing lower extremity function: Association with self-reported disability and prediction of mortality and nursing home admission. *J. Gerontol.* **1994**, *49*, M85–M94. [CrossRef] [PubMed]
16. Haskell, W.L.; Lee, I.-M.; Pate, R.R.; E Powell, K.; Blair, S.N.; A Franklin, B.; A Macera, C.; Heath, G.W.; Thompson, P.D.; Bauman, A.; et al. Physical activity and public health: Updated recommendation for adults from the American College of Sports Medicine and the American Heart Association. *Circulation* **2007**, *116*, 1081–1093. [CrossRef] [PubMed]
17. Haskell, W.L.; Lee, I.M.; Pate, R.R.; Powell, K.E.; Blair, S.N.; Franklin, B.A.; Macera, C.A.; Heath, G.W.; Thompson, P.D.; Bauman, A. Physical activity and public health: Updated recommendation for adults from the American College of Sports Medicine and the American Heart Association. *Med. Sci. Sports Exerc.* **2007**, *39*, 1423–1434. [CrossRef] [PubMed]
18. Poitras, V.J.; Gray, C.E.; Borghese, M.M.; Carson, V.; Chaput, J.-P.; Janssen, I.; Katzmarzyk, P.T.; Pate, R.R.; Connor Gorber, S.; Kho, M.E.; et al. Systematic review of the relationships between objectively measured physical activity and health indicators in school-aged children and youth. *Appl. Physiol. Nutr. Metab.* **2016**, *41*, S197–S239. [CrossRef]
19. Watson, A.; Dumuid, D.; Maher, C.; Olds, T. Associations between meeting 24-hour movement guidelines and academic achievement in Australian primary school-aged children. *J. Sport Health Sci.* **2022**, *11*, 521–529. [CrossRef] [PubMed]
20. Okely, A.D.; Ghersi, D.; Loughran, S.P.; Cliff, D.P.; Shilton, T.; Jones, R.A.; Stanley, R.M.; Sherring, J.; Toms, N.; Eckermann, S.; et al. A collaborative approach to adopting/adapting guidelines. The Australian 24-hour movement guidelines for children (5-12 years) and young people (13–17 years): An integration of physical activity, sedentary behaviour, and sleep. *Int. J. Behav. Nutr. Phys. Act.* **2022**, *19*, 2. [CrossRef]
21. Kline, C.E.; Hillman, C.H.; Sheppard, B.B.; Tennant, B.; Conroy, D.E.; Macko, R.F.; Marquez, D.X.; Petruzzello, S.J.; Powell, K.E.; Erickson, K.I. Physical activity and sleep: An updated umbrella review of the 2018 Physical Activity Guidelines Advisory Committee report. *Sleep Med. Rev.* **2021**, *58*, 101489. [CrossRef]
22. Cillekens, B.; Lang, M.; Van Mechelen, W.; Verhagen, E.; Huysmans, M.A.; Holtermann, A.; Van Der Beek, A.J.; Coenen, P. How does occupational physical activity influence health? An umbrella review of 23 health outcomes across 158 observational studies. *Br. J. Sports Med.* **2020**, *54*, 1474–1481. [CrossRef]
23. Sherrington, C.; Fairhall, N.J.; Wallbank, G.K.; Tiedemann, A.; A Michaleff, Z.; Howard, K.; Clemson, L.; Hopewell, S.; E Lamb, S. Exercise for preventing falls in older people living in the community. *Cochrane Database Syst. Rev.* **2019**, *1*, CD012424. [CrossRef]
24. Neefjes, E.C.; Hurk, R.M.V.D.; Blauwhoff-Buskermolen, S.; Van Der Vorst, M.J.; Becker-Commissaris, A.; De Van Der Schueren, M.A.; Buffart, L.M.; Verheul, H.M. Muscle mass as a target to reduce fatigue in patients with advanced cancer. *J. Cachex-Sarcopenia Muscle* **2017**, *8*, 623–629. [CrossRef] [PubMed]
25. Poole, D.C.; Burnley, M.; Vanhatalo, A.; Rossiter, H.B.; Jones, A.M. Critical Power: An Important Fatigue Threshold in Exercise Physiology. *Med. Sci. Sports Exerc.* **2016**, *48*, 2320–2334. [CrossRef] [PubMed]
26. Chen, L.-K.; Liu, L.-K.; Woo, J.; Assantachai, P.; Auyeung, T.-W.; Bahyah, K.S.; Chou, M.-Y.; Chen, L.-Y.; Hsu, P.-S.; Krairit, O.; et al. Sarcopenia in Asia: Consensus report of the Asian Working Group for Sarcopenia. *J. Am. Med. Dir. Assoc.* **2014**, *15*, 95–101. [CrossRef] [PubMed]
27. Kunutsor, S.K.; Leyland, S.; Skelton, D.A.; James, L.; Cox, M.; Gibbons, N.; Whitney, J.; Clark, E.M. Adverse events and safety issues associated with physical activity and exercise for adults with osteoporosis and osteopenia: A systematic review of observational studies and an updated review of interventional studies. *J. Frailty Sarcopenia Falls* **2018**, *3*, 155–178. [CrossRef]
28. Paluska, S.A.; Schwenk, T.L. Physical activity and mental health: Current concepts. *Sports Med.* **2000**, *29*, 167–180. [CrossRef]
29. Sankar, K.; Michael Christudhas, J.C. Influence of aging, disease, exercise, and injury on human hand movements: A systematic review. *Proc. Inst. Mech. Eng. Part H J. Eng. Med.* **2021**, *235*, 1221–1256. [CrossRef]
30. Matsui, N.; Miaki, H.; Kitagawa, T.; Nakagawa, T. Relationship between range of motion of foot joints and amount of physical activity in middle-aged male diabetic patients. *J. Phys. Ther. Sci.* **2019**, *31*, 540–544. [CrossRef]
31. Fox, K.R. The influence of physical activity on mental well-being. *Public Health Nutr.* **1999**, *2*, 411–418. [CrossRef]
32. Weyerer, S. Physical inactivity and depression in the community. Evidence from the Upper Bavarian Field Study. *Int. J. Sports Med.* **1992**, *13*, 492–496. [CrossRef]
33. Stephens, T. Physical activity and mental health in the United States and Canada: Evidence from four population surveys. *Prev. Med.* **1988**, *17*, 35–47. [CrossRef]
34. Thompson Coon, J.; Boddy, K.; Stein, K.; Whear, R.; Barton, J.; Depledge, M.H. Does participating in physical activity in outdoor natural environments have a greater effect on physical and mental wellbeing than physical activity indoors? A systematic review. *Environ. Sci. Technol.* **2011**, *45*, 1761–1772. [CrossRef] [PubMed]
35. Wunsch, K.; Kasten, N.; Fuchs, R. The effect of physical activity on sleep quality, well-being, and affect in academic stress periods. *Nat. Sci. Sleep* **2017**, *9*, 117–126. [CrossRef] [PubMed]
36. Nishiwaki, M.; Matsumoto, N. Physical activity and lifestyle intervention. *J. Phys. Fit. Sport. Med.* **2015**, *4*, 187–195. [CrossRef]
37. Bueno de Souza, R.O.; Marcon, L.F.; Arruda, A.S.F.; Pontes Junior, F.L.; Melo, R.C. Effects of Mat Pilates on Physical Functional Performance of Older Adults: A Meta-analysis of Randomized Controlled Trials. *Am. J. Phys. Med. Rehabilitation* **2018**, *97*, 414–425. [CrossRef]

38. Reimers, C.D.; Knapp, G.; Reimers, A.K. Does physical activity increase life expectancy? A review of the literature. *J. Aging Res.* **2012**, *2012*, 243958. [CrossRef]
39. Saint-Maurice, P.F.; Troiano, R.P.; Bassett, D.R.; Graubard, B.I.; Carlson, S.A.; Shiroma, E.J.; Fulton, J.E.; Matthews, C.E. Association of Daily Step Count and Step Intensity With Mortality Among US Adults. *JAMA* **2020**, *323*, 1151–1160. [CrossRef]
40. Friedenreich, C.M.; Stone, C.R.; Cheung, W.Y.; Hayes, S.C. Physical Activity and Mortality in Cancer Survivors: A Systematic Review and Meta-Analysis. *JNCI Cancer Spectr.* **2020**, *4*, pkz080. [CrossRef]
41. Costa, E.C.; Hay, J.L.; Kehler, D.S.; Boreskie, K.F.; Arora, R.C.; Umpierre, D.; Szwajcer, A.; Duhamel, T.A. Effects of High-Intensity Interval Training Versus Moderate-Intensity Continuous Training on Blood Pressure in Adults with Pre- to Established Hypertension: A Systematic Review and Meta-Analysis of Randomized Trials. *Sports Med.* **2018**, *48*, 2127–2142. [CrossRef]
42. Liu, Y.; Ye, W.; Chen, Q.; Zhang, Y.; Kuo, C.H.; Korivi, M. Resistance Exercise Intensity is Correlated with Attenuation of HbA1c and Insulin in Patients with Type 2 Diabetes: A Systematic Review and Meta-Analysis. *Int. J. Environ. Res. Public Health* **2019**, *16*, 140. [CrossRef]
43. Penedo, F.J.; Dahn, J.R. Exercise and well-being: A review of mental and physical health benefits associated with physical activity. *Curr. Opin. Psychiatry* **2005**, *18*, 189–193. [CrossRef]
44. Babyak, M.; Blumenthal, J.A.; Herman, S.; Khatri, P.; Doraiswamy, M.; Moore, K.; Craighead, W.E.; Baldewicz, T.T.; Krishnan, K.R. Exercise treatment for major depression: Maintenance of therapeutic benefit at 10 months. *Psychosom. Med.* **2000**, *62*, 633–638. [CrossRef] [PubMed]
45. Sallis, J.F.; Grossman, R.M.; Pinski, R.B.; Patterson, T.L.; Nader, P.R. The development of scales to measure social support for diet and exercise behaviors. *Prev. Med.* **1987**, *16*, 825–836. [CrossRef] [PubMed]
46. Janisse, H.C.; Nedd, D.; Escamilla, S.; Nies, M.A. Physical activity, social support, and family structure as determinants of mood among European-American and African-American women. *Women Health* **2004**, *39*, 101–116. [CrossRef] [PubMed]
47. Garber, C.E.; Blissmer, B.; Deschenes, M.R.; Franklin, B.A.; LaMonte, M.J.; Lee, I.-M.; Nieman, D.C.; Swain, D.P. American College of Sports Medicine position stand. Quantity and quality of exercise for developing and maintaining cardiorespiratory, musculoskeletal, and neuromotor fitness in apparently healthy adults: Guidance for prescribing exercise. *Med. Sci. Sport. Exerc.* **2011**, *43*, 1334–1359. [CrossRef]
48. Silverman, M.N.; Deuster, P.A. Biological mechanisms underlying the role of physical fitness in health and resilience. *Interface Focus* **2014**, *4*, 20140040. [CrossRef]
49. Elenkov, I.J.; Wilder, R.L.; Chrousos, G.P.; Vizi, E.S. The sympathetic nerve–an integrative interface between two supersystems: The brain and the immune system. *Pharmacol. Rev.* **2000**, *52*, 595–638.
50. Mastorakos, G.; Ilias, I. Interleukin-6: A cytokine and/or a major modulator of the response to somatic stress. *Ann. N. Y. Acad. Sci.* **2006**, *1088*, 373–381. [CrossRef]
51. Silverman, M.N.; Sternberg, E.M. Glucocorticoid regulation of inflammation and its functional correlates: From HPA axis to glucocorticoid receptor dysfunction. *Ann. N. Y. Acad. Sci.* **2012**, *1261*, 55–63. [CrossRef]
52. Banasr, M.; Duman, R.S. Regulation of neurogenesis and gliogenesis by stress and antidepressant treatment. *CNS Neurol. Disord.-Drug Targets* **2007**, *6*, 311–320. [CrossRef]
53. Cotman, C.W.; Berchtold, N.C.; Christie, L.A. Exercise builds brain health: Key roles of growth factor cascades and inflammation. *Trends Neurosci.* **2007**, *30*, 464–472. [CrossRef]
54. Wahlin-Larsson, B.; Carnac, G.; Kadi, F. The influence of systemic inflammation on skeletal muscle in physically active elderly women. *Age* **2014**, *36*, 9718. [CrossRef]
55. Ukena, C.; Mahfoud, F.; Kindermann, M.; Kindermann, I.; Bals, R.; Voors, A.A.; van Veldhuisen, D.J.; Böhm, M. The cardiopulmonary continuum systemic inflammation as 'common soil' of heart and lung disease. *Int. J. Cardiol.* **2010**, *145*, 172–176. [CrossRef] [PubMed]
56. Minakata, Y.; Sugino, A.; Kanda, M.; Ichikawa, T.; Akamatsu, K.; Koarai, A.; Hirano, T.; Nakanishi, M.; Sugiura, H.; Matsunaga, K.; et al. Reduced level of physical activity in Japanese patients with chronic obstructive pulmonary disease. *Respir. Investig.* **2014**, *52*, 41–48. [CrossRef] [PubMed]
57. Pitta, F.; Troosters, T.; Spruit, M.A.; Probst, V.S.; Decramer, M.; Gosselink, R. Characteristics of physical activities in daily life in chronic obstructive pulmonary disease. *Am. J. Respir. Crit. Care Med.* **2005**, *171*, 972–977. [CrossRef] [PubMed]
58. Garcia-Rio, F.; Rojo, B.; Casitas, R.; Lores, V.; Madero, R.; Romero, D.; Galera, R.; Villasante, C. Prognostic value of the objective measurement of daily physical activity in patients with COPD. *Chest* **2012**, *142*, 338–346. [CrossRef]
59. Waschki, B.; Kirsten, A.; Holz, O.; Müller, K.-C.; Meyer, T.; Watz, H.; Magnussen, H. Physical activity is the strongest predictor of all-cause mortality in patients with COPD: A prospective cohort study. *Chest* **2011**, *140*, 331–342. [CrossRef]
60. E Jones, S.; Maddocks, M.; Kon, S.; Canavan, J.L.; Nolan, C.M.; Clark, A.L.; I Polkey, M.; Man, W.D.-C. Sarcopenia in COPD: Prevalence, clinical correlates and response to pulmonary rehabilitation. *Thorax* **2015**, *70*, 213–218. [CrossRef]
61. Lehouck, A.; Boonen, S.; Decramer, M.; Janssens, W. COPD, bone metabolism, and osteoporosis. *Chest* **2011**, *139*, 648–657. [CrossRef]
62. Yohannes, A.M.; Alexopoulos, G.S. Depression and anxiety in patients with COPD. *Eur. Respir. Rev.* **2014**, *23*, 345–349. [CrossRef]
63. Venkatesan, P. GOLD COPD report: 2023 update. *Lancet Respir. Med.* **2022**, *11*, 18. [CrossRef]

64. Nakanishi, M.; Minakata, Y.; Tanaka, R.; Sugiura, H.; Kuroda, H.; Yoshida, M.; Yamamoto, N. Simple standard equation for daily step count in Japanese patients with chronic obstructive pulmonary disease. *Int. J. Chronic Obstr. Pulm. Dis.* **2019**, *14*, 1967–1977. [CrossRef] [PubMed]
65. Waschki, B.; Spruit, M.A.; Watz, H.; Albert, P.S.; Shrikrishna, D.; Groenen, M.; Smith, C.; Man, W.D.-C.; Tal-Singer, R.; Edwards, L.D.; et al. Physical activity monitoring in COPD: Compliance and associations with clinical characteristics in a multicenter study. *Respir. Med.* **2012**, *106*, 522–530. [CrossRef] [PubMed]
66. Tashiro, H.; Takahashi, K.; Tanaka, M.; Sadamatsu, H.; Kurihara, Y.; Tajiri, R.; Takamori, A.; Naotsuka, H.; Imaizumi, H.; Kimura, S.; et al. Skeletal muscle is associated with exercise tolerance evaluated by cardiopulmonary exercise testing in Japanese patients with chronic obstructive pulmonary disease. *Sci. Rep.* **2021**, *11*, 15862. [CrossRef] [PubMed]
67. Maddocks, M.; Shrikrishna, D.; Vitoriano, S.; Natanek, S.A.; Tanner, R.J.; Hart, N.; Kemp, P.R.; Moxham, J.; Polkey, M.I.; Hopkinson, N.S. Skeletal muscle adiposity is associated with physical activity, exercise capacity and fibre shift in COPD. *Eur. Respir. J.* **2014**, *44*, 1188–1198. [CrossRef] [PubMed]
68. Yoshida, M.; Hiramoto, T.; Moriwaki, A.; Osoreda, H.; Iwanaga, T.; Inoue, H. Impact of extrapulmonary comorbidities on physical activity in chronic obstructive pulmonary disease in Japan: A cross-sectional study. *PLoS ONE* **2022**, *17*, e0270836. [CrossRef]
69. Zigmond, A.S.; Snaith, R.P. The hospital anxiety and depression scale. *Acta Psychiatr. Scand.* **1983**, *67*, 361–370. [CrossRef]
70. Dueñas-Espín, I.; Demeyer, H.; Gimeno-Santos, E.; I Polkey, M.; Hopkinson, N.; A Rabinovich, R.; Dobbels, F.; Karlsson, N.; Troosters, T.; Garcia-Aymerich, J. Depression symptoms reduce physical activity in COPD patients: A prospective multicenter study. *Int. J. Chronic Obstr. Pulm. Dis.* **2016**, *11*, 1287–1295. [CrossRef]
71. Gimeno-Santos, E.; Frei, A.; Steurer-Stey, C.; de Batlle, J.; Rabinovich, R.A.; Raste, Y.; Hopkinson, N.S.; Polkey, M.I.; Van Remoortel, H.; Troosters, T.; et al. Determinants and outcomes of physical activity in patients with COPD: A systematic review. *Thorax* **2014**, *69*, 731–739. [CrossRef]
72. Garcia-Rio, F.; Lores, V.; Mediano, O.; Rojo, B.; Hernanz, A.; López-Collazo, E.; Alvarez-Sala, R. Daily physical activity in patients with chronic obstructive pulmonary disease is mainly associated with dynamic hyperinflation. *Am. J. Respir. Crit. Care Med.* **2009**, *180*, 506–512. [CrossRef]
73. Boström, P.; Wu, J.; Jedrychowski, M.P.; Korde, A.; Ye, L.; Lo, J.C.; Rasbach, K.A.; Boström, E.A.; Choi, J.H.; Long, J.Z.; et al. A PGC1-alpha-dependent myokine that drives brown-fat-like development of white fat and thermogenesis. *Nature* **2012**, *481*, 463–468. [CrossRef]
74. Timmons, J.A.; Baar, K.; Davidsen, P.K.; Atherton, P.J. Is irisin a human exercise gene? *Nature* **2012**, *488*, E9–E10. discussion E-1. [CrossRef] [PubMed]
75. Ijiri, N.; Kanazawa, H.; Asai, K.; Watanabe, T.; Hirata, K. Irisin, a newly discovered myokine, is a novel biomarker associated with physical activity in patients with chronic obstructive pulmonary disease. *Respirology* **2015**, *20*, 612–617. [CrossRef] [PubMed]
76. Sugiyama, Y.; Asai, K.; Yamada, K.; Kureya, Y.; Ijiri, N.; Watanabe, T.; Kanazawa, H.; Hirata, K. Decreased levels of irisin, a skeletal muscle cell-derived myokine, are related to emphysema associated with chronic obstructive pulmonary disease. *Int. J. Chronic Obstr. Pulm. Dis.* **2017**, *12*, 765–772. [CrossRef] [PubMed]
77. Tanaka, R.; Sugiura, H.; Yamada, M.; Ichikawa, T.; Koarai, A.; Fujino, N.; Yanagisawa, S.; Onodera, K.; Numakura, T.; Sato, K.; et al. Physical inactivity is associated with decreased growth differentiation factor 11 in chronic obstructive pulmonary disease. *Int. J. Chronic Obstr. Pulm. Dis.* **2018**, *13*, 1333–1342. [CrossRef]
78. Berry, M.J.; Rejeski, W.J.; Miller, M.E.; Adair, N.E.; Lang, W.; Foy, C.G.; Katula, J.A. A lifestyle activity intervention in patients with chronic obstructive pulmonary disease. *Respir. Med.* **2010**, *104*, 829–839. [CrossRef]
79. Wouters, E.F.; Wouters, B.B.; Augustin, I.M.; Houben-Wilke, S.; Vanfleteren, L.E.; Franssen, F.M. Personalised pulmonary rehabilitation in COPD. *Eur. Respir. Rev.* **2018**, *27*, 170125. [CrossRef]
80. Blackstock, F.C.; Lareau, S.C.; Nici, L.; ZuWallack, R.; Bourbeau, J.; Buckley, M.; Durning, S.J.; Effing, T.W.; Egbert, E.; Goldstein, R.S.; et al. Chronic Obstructive Pulmonary Disease Education in Pulmonary Rehabilitation. An Official American Thoracic Society/Thoracic Society of Australia and New Zealand/Canadian Thoracic Society/British Thoracic Society Workshop Report. *Ann. Am. Thorac. Soc.* **2018**, *15*, 769–784. [CrossRef]
81. Venkatesan, P. GOLD report: 2022 update. *Lancet Respir. Med.* **2022**, *10*, e20. [CrossRef]
82. Marengoni, A.; Vetrano, D.L.; Manes-Gravina, E.; Bernabei, R.; Onder, G.; Palmer, K. The Relationship Between COPD and Frailty: A Systematic Review and Meta-Analysis of Observational Studies. *Chest* **2018**, *154*, 21–40. [CrossRef]
83. Benz, E.; Trajanoska, K.; LaHousse, L.; Schoufour, J.D.; Terzikhan, N.; De Roos, E.; De Jonge, G.B.; Williams, R.; Franco, O.H.; Brusselle, G.; et al. Sarcopenia in COPD: A systematic review and meta-analysis. *Eur. Respir. Rev.* **2019**, *28*, 190049. [CrossRef]
84. Bolton, C.E.; Bevan-Smith, E.F.; Blakey, J.D.; Crowe, P.; Elkin, S.L.; Garrod, R.; Greening, N.J.; Heslop, K.; Hull, J.H.; Man, W.D.-C.; et al. British Thoracic Society guideline on pulmonary rehabilitation in adults. *Thorax* **2013**, *68* (Suppl. S2), ii1–ii30. [CrossRef]
85. Morris, N.R.; Hill, K.; Walsh, J.; Sabapathy, S. Exercise & Sports Science Australia (ESSA) position statement on exercise and chronic obstructive pulmonary disease. *J. Sci. Med. Sport* **2021**, *24*, 52–59. [CrossRef]
86. McCarthy, B.; Casey, D.; Devane, D.; Murphy, K.; Murphy, E.; Lacasse, Y. Pulmonary rehabilitation for chronic obstructive pulmonary disease. *Cochrane Database Syst. Rev.* **2015**, *2*, CD003793. [CrossRef] [PubMed]
87. Valeiro, B.; Rodríguez, E.; Pérez, P.; Gómez, A.; Mayer, A.I.; Pasarín, A.; Ibañez, J.; Ferrer, J.; Ramon, M.A. Promotion of physical activity after hospitalization for COPD exacerbation: A randomized control trial. *Respirology*, **2022**; *in press*. [CrossRef]

88. Maltais, F.; Leblanc, P.; Jobin, J.; Bérubé, C.; Bruneau, J.; Carrier, L.; Breton, M.J.; Falardeau, G.; Belleau, R. Intensity of training and physiologic adaptation in patients with chronic obstructive pulmonary disease. *Am. J. Respir. Crit. Care Med.* **1997**, *155*, 555–561. [CrossRef]
89. Jakobsson, J.; De Brandt, J.; Nyberg, A. Physiological responses and adaptations to exercise training in people with or without chronic obstructive pulmonary disease: Protocol for a systematic review and meta-analysis. *BMJ Open* **2022**, *12*, e065832. [CrossRef]
90. Kunik, M.E.; Roundy, K.; Veazey, C.; Souchek, J.; Richardson, P.; Wray, N.P.; Stanley, M.A. Surprisingly high prevalence of anxiety and depression in chronic breathing disorders. *Chest* **2005**, *127*, 1205–1211. [CrossRef] [PubMed]
91. Withers, N.J.; Rudkin, S.T.; White, R.J. Anxiety and depression in severe chronic obstructive pulmonary disease: The effects of pulmonary rehabilitation. *J. Cardiopulm. Rehabil.* **1999**, *19*, 362–365. [CrossRef] [PubMed]
92. Tremblay, M.S.; Aubert, S.; Barnes, J.D.; Saunders, T.J.; Carson, V.; Latimer-Cheung, A.E.; Chastin, S.F.M.; Altenburg, T.M.; Chinapaw, M.J.M.; on behalf of SBRN Terminology Consensus Project Participants. Sedentary Behavior Research Network (SBRN)—Terminology Consensus Project process and outcome. *Int. J. Behav. Nutr. Phys. Act.* **2017**, *14*, 75. [CrossRef] [PubMed]
93. Matthews, C.E.; Chen, K.Y.; Freedson, P.S.; Buchowski, M.S.; Beech, B.M.; Pate, R.R.; Troiano, R.P. Amount of time spent in sedentary behaviors in the United States, 2003–2004. *Am. J. Epidemiol.* **2008**, *167*, 875–881. [CrossRef]
94. Biswas, A.; Oh, P.I.; Faulkner, G.E.; Bajaj, R.R.; Silver, M.A.; Mitchell, M.S.; Alter, D.A. Sedentary time and its association with risk for disease incidence, mortality, and hospitalization in adults: A systematic review and meta-analysis. *Ann. Intern. Med.* **2015**, *162*, 123–132. [CrossRef] [PubMed]
95. Katzmarzyk, P.T.; Church, T.S.; Craig, C.L.; Bouchard, C. Sitting time and mortality from all causes, cardiovascular disease, and cancer. *Med. Sci. Sports Exerc.* **2009**, *41*, 998–1005. [CrossRef] [PubMed]
96. Healy, G.N.; Dunstan, D.W.; Salmon, J.; Cerin, E.; Shaw, J.E.; Zimmet, P.Z.; Owen, N. Objectively measured light-intensity physical activity is independently associated with 2-h plasma glucose. *Diabetes Care* **2007**, *30*, 1384–1389. [CrossRef] [PubMed]
97. Healy, G.N.; Wijndaele, K.; Dunstan, D.W.; Shaw, J.E.; Salmon, J.; Zimmet, P.Z.; Owen, N. Objectively measured sedentary time, physical activity, and metabolic risk: The Australian Diabetes, Obesity and Lifestyle Study (AusDiab). *Diabetes Care* **2008**, *31*, 369–371. [CrossRef]
98. Balkau, B.; Mhamdi, L.; Oppert, J.-M.; Nolan, J.; Golay, A.; Porcellati, F.; Laakso, M.; Ferrannini, E.; on behalf of the EGIR-RISC Study Group. Physical activity and insulin sensitivity: The RISC study. *Diabetes* **2008**, *57*, 2613–2618. [CrossRef]
99. Zerwekh, J.E.; Ruml, L.A.; Gottschalk, F.; Pak, C.Y.C. The effects of twelve weeks of bed rest on bone histology, biochemical markers of bone turnover, and calcium homeostasis in eleven normal subjects. *J. Bone Miner. Res.* **2009**, *13*, 1594–1601. [CrossRef]
100. Tremblay, M.S.; Colley, R.C.; Saunders, T.J.; Healy, G.N.; Owen, N. Physiological and health implications of a sedentary lifestyle. *Appl. Physiol. Nutr. Metab.* **2010**, *35*, 725–740. [CrossRef]
101. Hills, A.P.; Hennig, E.M.; Byrne, N.M.; Steele, J.R. The biomechanics of adiposity—Structural and functional limitations of obesity and implications for movement. *Obes. Rev.* **2002**, *3*, 35–43. [CrossRef]
102. Tremblay, M.S.; Willms, J.D. Is the Canadian childhood obesity epidemic related to physical inactivity? *Int. J. Obes.* **2003**, *27*, 1100–1105. [CrossRef]
103. Hu, F.B.; Li, T.Y.; Colditz, G.A.; Willett, W.C.; Manson, J.E. Television watching and other sedentary behaviors in relation to risk of obesity and type 2 diabetes mellitus in women. *JAMA* **2003**, *289*, 1785–1791. [CrossRef]
104. Brown, W.J.; Williams, L.; Ford, J.H.; Ball, K.; Dobson, A.J. Identifying the energy gap: Magnitude and determinants of 5-year weight gain in midage women. *Obes. Res.* **2005**, *13*, 1431–1441. [CrossRef]
105. Howard, R.A.; Freedman, D.M.; Park, Y.; Hollenbeck, A.; Schatzkin, A.; Leitzmann, M.F. Physical activity, sedentary behavior, and the risk of colon and rectal cancer in the NIH-AARP Diet and Health Study. *Cancer Causes Control.* **2008**, *19*, 939–953. [CrossRef] [PubMed]
106. Gierach, G.L.; Chang, S.C.; Brinton, L.A.; Lacey, J.V., Jr.; Hollenbeck, A.R.; Schatzkin, A.; Leitzmann, M.F. Physical activity, sedentary behavior, and endometrial cancer risk in the NIH-AARP Diet and Health Study. *Int. J. Cancer* **2009**, *124*, 2139–2147. [CrossRef] [PubMed]
107. Ford, E.S.; Caspersen, C.J. Sedentary behaviour and cardiovascular disease: A review of prospective studies. *Int. J. Epidemiol.* **2012**, *41*, 1338–1353. [CrossRef] [PubMed]
108. Dempsey, P.C.; Larsen, R.N.; Dunstan, D.W.; Owen, N.; Kingwell, B.A. Sitting Less and Moving More: Implications for Hypertension. *Hypertension* **2018**, *72*, 1037–1046. [CrossRef] [PubMed]
109. Wilmot, E.G.; Edwardson, C.L.; Achana, F.A.; Davies, M.J.; Gorely, T.; Gray, L.J.; Khunti, K.; Yates, T.; Biddle, S.J.H. Sedentary time in adults and the association with diabetes, cardiovascular disease and death: Systematic review and meta-analysis. *Diabetologia* **2012**, *55*, 2895–2905. [CrossRef] [PubMed]
110. Sanchez-Villegas, A.; Ara, I.; Guillen-Grima, F.; Bes-Rastrollo, M.; Varo-Cenarruzabeitia, J.J.; Martinez-Gonzalez, M.A. Physical activity, sedentary index, and mental disorders in the SUN cohort study. *Med. Sci. Sports Exerc.* **2008**, *40*, 827–834. [CrossRef]
111. Lei, Y.; Zou, K.; Xin, J.; Wang, Z.; Liang, K.; Zhao, L.; Ma, X. Sedentary behavior is associated with chronic obstructive pulmonary disease: A generalized propensity score-weighted analysis. *Medicine* **2021**, *100*, e25336. [CrossRef]
112. O'Donnell, D.E.; Webb, K.A. Exertional breathlessness in patients with chronic airflow limitation. The role of lung hyperinflation. *Am. Rev. Respir. Dis.* **1993**, *148*, 1351–1357. [CrossRef]

113. O'Donnell, D.E.; Revill, S.M.; Webb, K.A. Dynamic hyperinflation and exercise intolerance in chronic obstructive pulmonary disease. *Am. J. Respir. Crit. Care Med.* **2001**, *164*, 770–777. [CrossRef]
114. Tashiro, H.; Kurihara, Y.; Takahashi, K.; Sadamatsu, H.; Haraguchi, T.; Tajiri, R.; Takamori, A.; Kimura, S.; Sueoka-Aragane, N. Clinical features of Japanese patients with exacerbations of chronic obstructive pulmonary disease. *BMC Pulm. Med.* **2020**, *20*, 318. [CrossRef] [PubMed]
115. Horita, N.; Kaneko, T.; Shinkai, M.; Yomota, M.; Morita, S.; Rubin, B.K.; Ishigatsubo, Y. Depression in Japanese patients with chronic obstructive pulmonary disease: A cross-sectional study. *Respir. Care* **2013**, *58*, 1196–1203. [CrossRef] [PubMed]
116. Minakata, Y.; Motegi, T.; Ueki, J.; Gon, Y.; Nakamura, S.; Anzai, T.; Hirata, K.; Ichinose, M. Effect of tiotropium/olodaterol on sedentary and active time in patients with COPD: Post hoc analysis of the VESUTO((R)) study. *Int. J. Chronic Obstr. Pulm. Dis.* **2019**, *14*, 1789–1801. [CrossRef] [PubMed]
117. Takahashi, K.; Uchida, M.; Kato, G.; Takamori, A.; Kinoshita, T.; Yoshida, M.; Tajiri, R.; Kojima, K.; Inoue, H.; Kobayashi, H.; et al. First-Line Treatment with Tiotropium/Olodaterol Improves Physical Activity in Patients with Treatment-Naive Chronic Obstructive Pulmonary Disease. *Int. J. Chronic Obstr. Pulm. Dis.* **2020**, *15*, 2115–2126. [CrossRef]
118. Takahashi, K.; Tashiro, H.; Tajiri, R.; Takamori, A.; Uchida, M.; Kato, G.; Kurihara, Y.; Sadamatsu, H.; Kinoshita, T.; Yoshida, M.; et al. Factors Associated with Reduction of Sedentary Time Following Tiotropium/Olodaterol Therapy in Treatment-Naive Chronic Obstructive Pulmonary Disease. *Int. J. Chronic Obstr. Pulm. Dis.* **2021**, *16*, 3297–3307. [CrossRef]
119. Rabe, K.F.; Martinez, F.J.; Ferguson, G.T.; Wang, C.; Singh, D.; Wedzicha, J.A.; Trivedi, R.; Rose, E.S.; Ballal, S.; McLaren, J.; et al. Triple Inhaled Therapy at Two Glucocorticoid Doses in Moderate-to-Very-Severe COPD. *N. Engl. J. Med.* **2020**, *383*, 35–48. [CrossRef]
120. Breyer, M.-K.; Breyer-Kohansal, R.; Funk, G.-C.; Dornhofer, N.; A Spruit, M.; Wouters, E.F.; Burghuber, O.C.; Hartl, S. Nordic walking improves daily physical activities in COPD: A randomised controlled trial. *Respir. Res.* **2010**, *11*, 112. [CrossRef]
121. Vasilopoulou, M.; Papaioannou, A.I.; Kaltsakas, G.; Louvaris, Z.; Chynkiamis, N.; Spetsioti, S.; Kortianou, E.; Genimata, S.A.; Palamidas, A.; Kostikas, K.; et al. Home-based maintenance tele-rehabilitation reduces the risk for acute exacerbations of COPD, hospitalisations and emergency department visits. *Eur. Respir. J.* **2017**, *49*, 1602129. [CrossRef]
122. Wootton, S.L.; Hill, K.; Alison, J.A.; Ng, L.W.C.; Jenkins, S.; Eastwood, P.R.; Hillman, D.R.; Jenkins, C.; Spencer, L.; Cecins, N.; et al. Effects of ground-based walking training on daily physical activity in people with COPD: A randomised controlled trial. *Respir. Med.* **2017**, *132*, 139–145. [CrossRef]
123. Cruz, J.; Brooks, D.; Marques, A. Walk2Bactive: A randomised controlled trial of a physical activity-focused behavioural intervention beyond pulmonary rehabilitation in chronic obstructive pulmonary disease. *Chronic Respir. Dis.* **2016**, *13*, 57–66. [CrossRef]
124. Cheng, S.W.M.; Alison, J.; Stamatakis, E.; Dennis, S.; McNamara, R.; Spencer, L.; McKeough, Z. Six-week behaviour change intervention to reduce sedentary behaviour in people with chronic obstructive pulmonary disease: A randomised controlled trial. *Thorax* **2022**, *77*, 231–238. [CrossRef] [PubMed]

Disclaimer/Publisher's Note: The statements, opinions and data contained in all publications are solely those of the individual author(s) and contributor(s) and not of MDPI and/or the editor(s). MDPI and/or the editor(s) disclaim responsibility for any injury to people or property resulting from any ideas, methods, instructions or products referred to in the content.

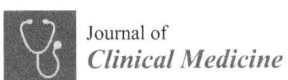

Review

Objective Measurement of Physical Activity and Sedentary Behavior in Patients with Chronic Obstructive Pulmonary Disease: Points to Keep in Mind during Evaluations

Yoshiaki Minakata *, Yuichiro Azuma, Seigo Sasaki and Yusuke Murakami

National Hospital Organization Wakayama Hospital, 1138 Wada, Mihama-Cho, Hidaka-gun, Wakayama 644-0044, Japan; azuma19841025@yahoo.co.jp (Y.A.); sasaki.seigo.su@mail.hosp.go.jp (S.S.); murakami.yusuke.am@mail.hosp.go.jp (Y.M.)
* Correspondence: minakata.yoshiaki.qy@mail.hosp.go.jp; Tel.: +81-738-22-3256

Abstract: Objective measurement methods using accelerometers have become the mainstream approach for evaluating physical activity (PA) and sedentary behavior (SB). However, several problems face the objective evaluation of PA and SB in patients with chronic obstructive pulmonary disease (COPD). For example, indicators of PA differ depending on whether the accelerometer detects the kind of activity on the one hand, or its intensity on the other. Measured data are also strongly influenced by environmental factors (weather, season, employment status, etc.) and methodological factors (days with uncommon activities, non-wearing time, minimum required wearing time per day, minimum number of valid days required, etc.). Therefore, adjusting for these factors is required when evaluating PA or SB, especially when evaluating the effects of intervention. The exclusion of sleeping time, unification of total measurement time, and minimization of the required wearing time per day might be more important for the evaluation of ST than for evaluating PA. The lying-down-time-to-sitting-time ratio was shown to be larger in COPD patients than in healthy subjects. In this review, we clarified the problems encountered during objective evaluations of PA and SB in patients with COPD and encouraged investigators to recognize the presence of these problems and the importance of adjusting for them.

Keywords: accelerometer; indicator; environmental factor; methodology; reproducibility

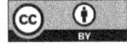

1. Introduction

Chronic obstructive pulmonary disease (COPD) is now a major cause of morbidity and mortality worldwide [1,2], and its burden is projected to increase in the coming decades because of continued exposure to COPD risk factors and the aging of the world's population [3]. Physical activity (PA) is lower in COPD patients than in healthy subjects [4,5] (Figure 1). A reduced level of PA was associated with a decline in forced expiratory volume in one second (FEV1) [6–10], COPD exacerbation [11–15], and mortality [11,16,17]. Furthermore, lower PA has been shown to be the strongest predictor of all-cause mortality in patients with COPD [17].

In COPD, hyperinflation causes exertional dyspnea, leading to a vicious cycle of a reduced exercise capacity, decreased PA, skeletal muscle dysfunction, and further dyspnea, thereby equating to a poor prognosis [18]. Exercise capacity reflects a patient's maximal ability to do exercise, while PA reflects a patient's willingness to move. PA is defined as any bodily movement by skeletal muscle that results in energy expenditure [19] but is usually taken to mean physically active behavior that is comparable to moderate-to-vigorous-intensity PA (MVPA) [20,21].

The two parameters of "physical inactivity" and "sedentary behavior (SB)" are also considered when evaluating a subject's physical condition. Physical inactivity is defined as a PA level that is not sufficient for meeting present PA recommendations, which is

150 min of MVPA per week or 75 min of vigorous-intensity PA per week, or an equivalent combination of moderate- and vigorous-intensity activity [21,22]. Physical inactivity is simply the opposite of PA. SB is defined as any waking behavior characterized by an energy expenditure ≤1.5 metabolic equivalents (METs) while in a sitting, reclining, or lying-down posture [21,23,24]. As SB is a risk factor for COPD mortality independently of PA [25], it has been attracting an increasing amount of attention in recent years [25–31].

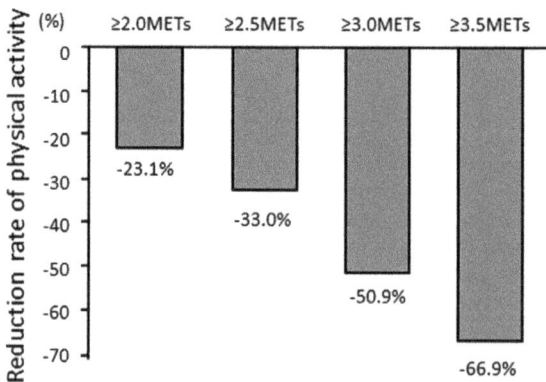

Figure 1. Mean reduction rate of PA in COPD patients compared to healthy subjects. Mean reduction rate of PA in COPD patients was calculated as 100 × [(mean duration of PA in COPD) − (mean duration of PA in healthy subjects)]/(mean duration of PA in healthy subjects) at each intensity of PA. PA: physical activity; COPD: Chronic obstructive pulmonary disease; METs: metabolic equivalents. Quoted from reference [5].

Objective measurement methods using accelerometers have become mainstream approaches for evaluating PA and SB, replacing conventional questionnaire-based methods, which tended to overestimate the findings [32]. However, objective approaches still involve several issues that remain to be resolved. While data obtained by objective measurements are thought to be highly accurate, no adjusting for influencing factors can reduce the reliability and significantly affect results, especially in intervention studies. Furthermore, PA is behavior with a relatively high intensity and accounts for only a small part of the day, whereas SB has a low intensity and accounts for most of our waking hours. This should be kept in mind when evaluating PA or SB with an accelerometer.

In this narrative review, we clarified the problems encountered during objective evaluations for PA and SB in patients with COPD and encouraged investigators to recognize the presence of these problems and the importance of adjusting for them.

2. The Objective Measurement of PA in COPD

2.1. Self-Reported vs. Objectively Measured PA

When the duration at ≥2.0 METs measured by a questionnaire and that by an accelerometer were compared in COPD patients, most of the patients showed higher values based on a questionnaire than based on an accelerometer evaluation (Figure 2), and the mean (±standard deviation [SD]) values were 366.7 (221.8) min and 201.2 (99.1) min, respectively [32]. When the duration at >3.0 METs measured by a questionnaire and that by an accelerometer were compared, these values were 146 (143.1) min and 65 (89.4) min, respectively [33]. A systematic review showed that self-reported assessments overestimate the level of PA compared with objectively measured assessments [34]. Therefore, the objectively measured assessments are accurate, although they have various technical and associated difficulties.

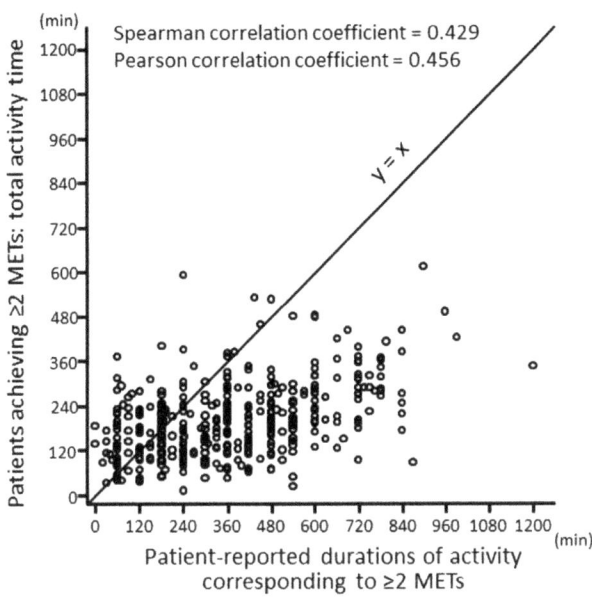

Figure 2. Correlations between objectively measured and patient-reported durations of PA equivalent to ≥2 METs. PA: physical activity; METs: metabolic equivalents. Quoted from reference [32] with permission.

2.2. Types of Accelerometry

Accelerometers are roughly classified into two types: those that detect the kinds of activity undertaken (e.g., DynaPort MoveMonitor™ from McRobert BV, the Hague, The Netherlands) and those that detect the intensity of activity (e.g., SenseWear Armband™ from BodyMedia Inc., Pittsburgh, PA, USA; Active Style Pro HJA-750C™ from Omron Health Care, Kyoto, Japan; etc.). Both types of accelerometers can measure total PA and the daily step count. In the type that detects intensity of activity, the results are expressed as acceleration for some models and activity intensity for others.

2.3. Indicators

There are various indicators for assessing PA, depending on the type of accelerometer used. When accelerometers that detect kinds of activity are used, the duration of walking and/or standing, proportion of the duration of walking and/or standing to that of total activity, movement intensity during movement, and total step count can be used as indicators. When accelerometers that detect intensity of activity are used, durations of several intensities, e.g., light PA (LPA; 1.5–3.0 METs), moderate PA (MPA; 3.0–6.0 METs), vigorous PA (VPA; ≥6.0 METs), moderate-to-vigorous PA (MVPA; ≥3.0 METs), LPA + MVPA (≥2.0 METs), total PA at ≥3.0 METs (METs·h), and step count can be used as indicators. Some accelerometers display the results in acceleration intensity rather than activity intensity. The values for these metrics are evaluated daily or weekly.

2.4. Validated Accelerometers for COPD

Regarding accelerometers that detect the kind of activity undertaken, the DynaPort Activity Monitor™ (McRoberts BV) [4], which is the old version of the DynaPort MoveMonitor™, and the new DynaPort MoveMonitor™ [35–37] are validated for use in COPD patients. Regarding accelerometers that detect the intensity of activity, the SenseWear Armband™ (Bodymedia Inc.) [34,35,37,38], RT3™ (StayHealthy Inc., Monrovia, CA, USA) [35,37,39], Actiwatch Spectrum™ (Philips Respironics, Bend, OR, USA) [35,37],

Actigraph GT3X™ (Actigraph LLC, Pensacola, FL, USA) [37,40], Lifecorder™ (Kenz Suzuken Co. Ltd., Nagoya, Japan) [35,37], Actimarker™ (Panasonic, Osaka, Japan) [41], and Active Style Pro HJA-750C™ [42] have been validated for use in COPD patients.

While pedometers tended to detect low step counts for slow-walking people such as those with COPD [43], triaxial accelerometers including the DynaPort™ [44], SenseWear Armband™ [45], and Actigraph GT3X™ [46] have been able to detect slow walking. Furthermore, the Active Style Pro HJA-750C™ uses different algorithms for two different kinds of activities (household and locomotive activities), so it may be more useful for monitoring COPD patients, who often engage in low-intensity activity [47,48].

2.5. Environmental Factors Requiring Adjustments for Evaluations

Environmental factors can influence the PA level. These factors should be included in the individual's average PA level, but they can also influence the results when comparing changes in PA over time. As these factors can lead to intra-patient errors, they should be minimized for longitudinal evaluations.

2.5.1. Weather

Weather is one such environmental factor. The duration of PA and step count are significantly reduced on rainy days in comparison to non-rainy days [41,42,49–51]. Indeed, the duration of PA at ≥ 3.0 METs was shown to be 11.1 min on rainy days and 21.3 min on non-rainy days [41]. Furthermore, the daily step count was 3999 on non-rainy days and 3771 on rainy days [49], although this difference was below the minimal clinically important difference. Rainfall of 10 mm translated to a decrease of approximately 175 steps [50].

2.5.2. Season

Season is another potential environmental factor, as the duration of PA is longer in summer than in winter [52–54]. Temperature might be the main factor associated with these seasonal effects. For example, when the average temperature was ≤ 20.5 °C, more COPD patients went out as the temperatures became warmer (odds ratio [OR]: 1.028 per 1 °C rise in temperature), and at <2.5 °C, the increase in patients going outdoors with rising temperature grew significantly (OR: 1.13 per 1 °C rise). However, when the temperature was >20.5 °C, patients reduced outdoor activity (OR: 0.96 per 1 °C rise) [55]. When the average temperature was ≤ 22.5 °C, the daily step count increased 43 steps per 1 °C rise, and at >22.5 °C, the daily step count fell by 891 steps per 1 °C increase in temperature [49]. The daily step count increased 316 steps for each 10 °C rise in temperature [50]. The duration of daylight time may also influence PA [52].

2.5.3. Day of the Week

The day of the week might also influence PA. The PA on weekends was shown to be reduced compared to weekdays in healthy subjects [56–58]. However, the PA on weekends was not significantly different from that on weekdays in COPD patients [39,42]. Most healthy subjects were working, while most COPD patients were retired. The level of PA in patients with a job is higher than in those without a job [32]. Therefore, when PA is investigated in retired COPD patients, the timing of weekends or holidays might not need to be taken into consideration.

2.5.4. Air Pollution

Air pollution might influence PA. In one report, the time spent outdoors decreased with increasing ozone levels but not with PM10 values. An increased ozone level decreased both the time spent outdoors and daily step count [49]. In another report, however, PA was not correlated with the values of main atmospheric pollutants, including PM10, ozone, nitrogen dioxide, and sulfur dioxide [51]. The effects of air pollution on PA are therefore still controversial.

2.5.5. Employment Status

Employment status can also influence PA. The duration at ≥ 3.0 METs and step count in non-employed patients were significantly lower than in employed patients according to a multivariate analysis (-13.2 ± 2.9 min and -1332.3 ± 295.6 steps, respectively, compared to employed patients) [32]. Most COPD patients seem to be retired, but caution should be practiced when evaluating subjects who have a job.

2.6. Methodological Factors Requiring Adjustments for Evaluations
2.6.1. Days with Uncommon Activities

In our daily lives, there are days when we engage in relatively uncommon activities, such as traveling or recuperating from sickness. Data from days spent engaged in these uncommon activities are therefore not representative of the usual PA and should be excluded from the analysis.

2.6.2. Non-Wearing Time

Even if the subject is active, the measurement result will show inactivity if the accelerometer is not worn. Therefore, the detection of non-wear time is an important issue when measuring PA using an accelerometer. For accelerometers that can be attached directly to the skin of the arm to collect biometric information, such as a SenseWear™ or Actiwatch™, it is possible to detect non-wearing. However, these models are relatively expensive, and as most other accelerometers cannot collect biological information, it is necessary to set detecting conditions for non-wearing.

PA below the detection limit of the accelerometer (e.g., 1.0 METs) also cannot be measured, but most reports refer to non-measurement time as non-wearing time. In such cases, there is a risk of resting behavior being considered non-wearing time. In some studies, a non-measurement time of 60 consecutive minutes has been defined as non-wearing time [59]. Recently, a more precise definition of non-wearing time was used for COPD patients, consisting of 90 consecutive minutes of non-measurement time with an allowance of 2 min of interruption [60,61].

2.6.3. Minimum Required Wearing Time per Day

In previous reports, most studies reported findings without assessing the actual wearing time [62]. Demeyer et al. recommended a wearing time of at least 8 h [63], and the minimum wearing times used were 8 [32,64–66], 12 [67], or 20 h [68].

2.6.4. Minimum Number of Valid Days Required

Even after adjusting for environmental and methodological factors, the amount of daily activity can easily change from day to day. Generally, one's representative PA value is calculated as the average or sum of daily PA values over a certain period of time. Therefore, the minimum number of days required to obtain repeatability should be determined. The repeatability has been evaluated using intraclass correlation coefficients, and the number of days of measurements required in COPD patients has ranged from two to seven [62]. Watz et al. reported that a minimum of two to three days was required in stage IV COPD patients, whereas it was five days in stage I COPD patients [69]. Demeyer et al. recommended measuring for at least four weekdays when assessing step and light activity with a Sensewear Armband™ [63]. After adjusting for environmental and methodological factors, the minimum number of days required to obtain reproducibility was three for both the Actimarker™ [41] and Active Style Pro HJA-750C™ [42].

2.7. Patient Conditions Influencing PA

PA in COPD patients can be influenced by several patient factors, including demographic factors, the pulmonary function, dyspnea, exercise capacity, comorbidities, muscular conditions, mental state, and living environment. These factors can lead to inter-patient differences in PA, but the associations are still controversial at present.

The age [5,32,70,71], dyspnea [5,32,70–74], exercise capacity [5,71–73], and pulmonary function—including FEV1 [5,32,71,72,75], inspiratory capacity (IC) [70,76], and diffusing capacity [5,73]—are all important factors potentially influencing PA in COPD patients. Depression [75,77], cardiac dysfunction [71], dog walking, grandparenting [78], and employment status [32] can also influence PA in COPD patients.

Muscle quality may also be a relevant factor influencing PA. Muscle mass, especially the cross-sectional area of the erector spine muscle assessed by chest computed tomography (ESM_{CSA}) [79], and muscle strength, especially the quadriceps strength [72,80], were shown to be associated with PA in COPD patients. Myokines, especially irisin [81] and growth differentiation factor 11 [82], have been reported to be associated with PA in COPD patients.

Regarding serological tests, C-reactive protein (CRP), fibrinogen, and interleukin-6 values were reported to be associated with PA in COPD patients [78,83,84]. In another report, however, the CRP value was not associated with PA [85]. Furthermore, Taka et al. reported that SIRT1 and FOXO1 mRNA might be associated with PA in COPD patients [86].

2.8. Interventions for Improving PA

Evidence concerning the improvement in PA with interventions, including pharmacological management and pulmonary rehabilitation, has been limited, possibly due to a lack of established methodological details, including optimal timing, components, duration, and models for interventions, as well as the evaluation methods. There has also been scant evidence supporting a continued effect over time after the end of intervention [87].

2.8.1. Pharmacological Interventions

Bronchodilator administration has been shown to improve PA in some reports [66,88–94], albeit depending on the indicator in some cases [95–97], while no improvement was seen in other reports [98–101]. When adjusted for at least two influencing factors, bronchodilators invariably showed beneficial effects on PA with some indicators [66,89–91,93,96,97]. However, none of the studies reporting that bronchodilators exerted no beneficial effect on PA performed such adjustments [98–101]. Consideration of potentially influential factors should therefore be required when evaluating the effects of intervention, and bronchodilators may thus yet be found to improve PA in all COPD patients [18]. Furthermore, when a long-acting muscarinic antagonist (LAMA) and a long-acting beta 2 adrenergic agonist (LABA)/LAMA combination agent were compared in a meta-analysis, PA was found to be significantly improved with LABA/LAMA treatment compared to LAMA [102].

2.8.2. Non-Pharmacological Interventions

Evidence supporting improvements in PA in COPD patients with pulmonary rehabilitation is also limited [87]. However, changes in PA with pulmonary rehabilitation combined with counseling using pedometer feedback have tended to be high [103]. Counseling is predominantly based on the principle of goal-setting and implementation of that goal [104,105]. A positive effect of providing target step count values using an internet-mediated program was seen after 3 or 4 months [106,107] but not after 12 months [108]. The disappearance of this effect after 12 months might have been because even if the patients worked hard to increase the number of steps taken each day, the target value was reviewed and then increased further each week; furthermore, the target value was set according to the current step count without considering the disease condition of each patient. These issues may have made it difficult for patients to remain motivated for a long time. Indeed, half of the participants believed the automated target step counts were too high, and many did not feel comfortable reaching their targets [109].

We created referent equations for step count using PA-associated factors for COPD patients (Figure 3) [70,71] and developed a method to set an individual target step count using the current steps and the steps calculated by the equation [110]. Furthermore, a pilot study found that providing a target value was able to increase the step count in patients with innately low step counts [110]. Although an intervention study conducted over a longer duration is required, this target value setting method reflecting the disease condition might be useful for increasing PA in COPD patients.

Simple Equation

Step count (steps) = (−0.079 × [age] − 1.595 × [mMRC] + 2.078*[IC] + 18.149) [3]

- -

Detailed Equations

Step count (steps) = (0.010 × [6MWD] − 0.666 × [mMRC] + 0.155 × [HADS-A] + 0.029 × [FEV1 %pred] + 9.843) [3]

Duration at ≥2.0METs (min) = (0.0010 × [6MWD] − 0.174 × [mMRC] + 0.055 × [HADS-A] + 0.0083 × [FEV1 %pred] + 4.973) [3]

Duration at ≥3.0METs (min) = (0.0017 × [6MWD] − 0.210 × [mMRC] + 0.037 × [HADS-A] + 0.0090 × [FEV1 %pred] − 0.015 × [age] + 3.764) [3]

Total activity at ≥3.0METs (METs*h) = (0.00067 × [6MWD] − 0.078 × [mMRC] + 0.016 × [HADS-A] + 0.0033 × [FEV1 %pred] − 0.00067 × [BNP] + 1.0013) [3]

Figure 3. Reference equations of PA using associated factors for COPD patients. PA: physical activity; COPD: chronic obstructive pulmonary disease; mMRC: modified Medical Research Council dyspnea scale; IC: inspiratory capacity; 6MWD: 6-minute walk distance; HADS-A: anxiety score of the Hospital Anxiety and Depression Scale; FEV1%pred: forced expiratory volume in one second percent of predicted value; BNP: serum brain natriuretic peptide. Quoted from references [67,68].

3. The Objective Measurement of SB in COPD

3.1. Sedentary Time (ST) in Subjects with Several Conditions

SB is defined as any waking behavior characterized by an energy expenditure ≤1.5 metabolic equivalents (METs) while in a sitting, reclining, or lying-down posture [21,23,24]. ST is one of the frequently used indicators of SB. The concept of ST has been attracting attention in the general population [111–116] as well as in patients with cardiovascular disease [117–119], diabetes mellitus [118,120,121], and cancer [112,122–126] because of our increasing awareness of our health condition and mortality risk. In COPD patients, ST was reported to be an independent predictor of mortality after adjusting for the duration at ≥3.0 METs and several other variables [25].

3.2. Objectively Measured ST and Its Problems

While an accelerometer might detect ST more precisely than a questionnaire, it is difficult to extract the exact ST according to the definition. Investigators should thus treat ST more carefully than PA, as ST accounts for more than half of the total measurement time and does not include the time spent moving during sleep. Associated issues with its measurement can include functional limitations of accelerometers, the exclusion of sleeping time, unification of the total measurement time per day, and minimum required wearing time.

3.2.1. Functional Limitations of Accelerometers

When an accelerometer that detects the kind of activity is used, the sitting time or sitting + lying-down time is employed as an indicator of ST. In such cases, however, the duration of behavior with an intensity of >1.5 METs while sitting, which is not SB, is included. In our investigation, such instances accounted for 27.5% of the sitting time [127]. Furthermore, the duration spent sleeping while sitting or lying down is also included. These times should be excluded from ST according to the definition (Figure 4) [18]. When an accelerometer that detects the intensity of activity is used, the duration of behavior with an intensity of 1.0–1.5 METs (including both 1.0 and 1.5 METs) [23,66,128] or the ratio of the duration of behavior at 1.0–1.5 METs to the total measurement time may be employed as indicators of ST. In such cases, however, the duration of behavior with an intensity of <1.0 METs is not included in the ST, as it cannot be detected by most accelerometers. Furthermore, the duration spent sleeping while still performing activity with an intensity of 1.0–1.5 METs is also included (Figure 4). These errors are functional limitations of the accelerometer and cannot be avoided. However, while an accurate measurement of ST by definition is difficult regardless of the type of accelerometer used, investigators need to aware that these errors exist and be prepared to compensate for them.

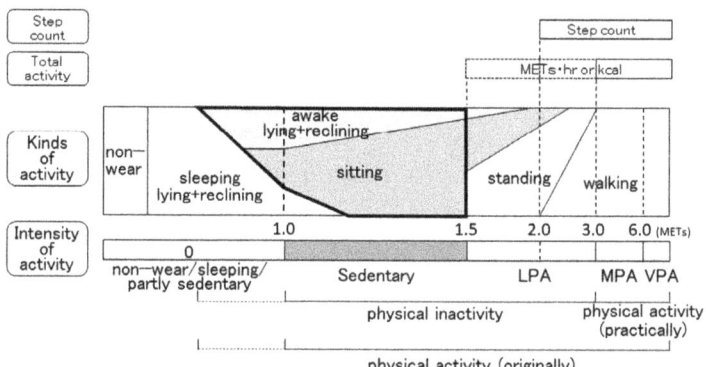

Figure 4. Indicators regarding the physical status based on a comparison of the intensity and kind of activity in cases of COPD. The area surrounded by a bold line indicates sedentary behavior according to the established definition. METs, metabolic equivalents; LPA, light-intensity physical activity; MPA, moderate-intensity physical activity; VPA, vigorous-intensity physical activity.

3.2.2. Exclusion of Sleeping Time

Exclusion of sleeping time is another problem for precisely detecting ST. Most behavior during sleep is <1.0 METs in intensity, but during some periods, it can reach ≥1.0 METs, which is incorrectly counted as ST. Furthermore, napping time is difficult to exclude. Since these times cannot be distinguished based on the results obtained with an accelerometer, investigators should keep this error in mind.

3.2.3. Unification of Total Measurement Time per Day

ST can be markedly affected by the total measurement time, as the time spent sitting and lying down accounts for 64% of the total measurement time in COPD patients [4]. Furthermore, subjects tend to feel less of a need to wear accelerometers when they are not active, which might lead to both the total measurement time and ST being shorter than the actual active time. It is therefore best to unify the measurement time if possible.

In some reports, subjects were instructed to wear an accelerometer from the time they woke up to the time they went to bed in order to exclude time spent sleeping [128–130]. However, these times varied from day to day and person to person, so the total measurement time varied among measurements. If subjects are instructed to wear an accelerometer at a particular time, such as from 6:00 am to 9:00 pm, some subjects may not have woken up yet at 6:00 am or may have already gone to bed at 9:00 pm. It might therefore be better to ask subjects to wear the accelerometer constantly and extract only the data for a defined period from all of the data obtained [28,66,131]. However, this method has the disadvantage of increasing the burden on the subject due to unnecessary data acquisition during sleep. There is no perfect method for unifying measurement times, so investigators should interpret the data with an understanding of the weaknesses associated with each method.

3.2.4. Minimum Required Wearing Time per Day

Even if the measurement time is unified, wearing time will decrease due to bathing or forgetting to wear the accelerometer. ST can be more strongly influenced by the wearing time than the duration of PA, simply because ST accounts for the majority of the measurement time. The minimum required wearing time was reported to be set to 8 [31], 10 [130,132–134], or 12 h [67,128,131,135] in previous studies, and the wearing time tended to be longer for SB assessments than for PA assessments. Further research is needed to confirm the optimal wearing time for evaluating ST.

3.3. Lying-Down-Time-to-Sitting-Time Ratio (LSR) in COPD Patients

Both the sitting and lying-down (including reclining) times are included in ST, and both set a lower levels in ST measured in COPD patients compared to those in healthy subjects [4]. However, when the lying-down time was compared with the sitting time, the LSR was larger in COPD patients (23.1%) than in healthy subjects (9.5%) [4]. We investigated the lying-down time and sitting time in COPD patients wearing both intensity-based and activity type-based accelerometers at the same time. The lying-down time accounted for 28.3% of the total wearing time (212 $\pm$ 160 min), and the sitting time accounted for 49.4% of the total wearing time (370 $\pm$ 123 min), resulting in the LSR being 57.3% [127]. Patients with COPD might spend more time lying down than expected during ST. Furthermore, the duration spent engaged in behaviors at 0 METs, 1.0–1.5 METs, and $\geq$3.0 METs while sitting accounted for 9.2%, 63.3%, and 27.5% of total time, respectively, and the duration spent engaged in those behaviors while lying down accounted for 29.5%, 62.7%, and 7.8%, respectively [127]. While we have previously described the relationship between the indicators measured with an intensity-based accelerometer and those with an activity type-based accelerometer [18], slight modifications are needed in cases of COPD, as shown in Figure 4.

3.4. Interventions for Improving ST

Since no objective measurement method has yet been established, few reports have demonstrated clear intervention effects. We sub-analyzed the results of a crossover study after strictly adjusting for factors affecting the ST and found that the LAMA/LABA combination significantly reduced the ST compared to LAMA alone [66]. This effect was confirmed in a meta-analysis, although the number of reports was only two [102]. Further research with strict adjustment for the influential factors will be required to clarify the effects of interventions.

4. Conclusions

The objective measurement of PA and SB is a promising method for clarifying the physical condition of COPD patients; however, several problems remain to be solved. Researchers need to recognize the existence of these problems and the importance of adjusting for them when evaluating.

Author Contributions: Y.M. (Yoshiaki Minakata): conceptualization, writing—original draft preparation, writing—review and editing; Y.A., S.S. and Y.M. (Yusuke Murakami): writing—original draft preparation, writing—review and editing. All authors have read and agreed to the published version of the manuscript.

Funding: This research was funded by the Environmental Restoration and Conservation Agency of Japan, Funding number : None. URL: https://www.erca.go.jp/yobou/zensoku/investigate/ (accessed on 30 March 2023).

Institutional Review Board Statement: Not applicable.

Informed Consent Statement: Not applicable.

Data Availability Statement: Not applicable.

Acknowledgments: The authors thank Brian Quinn for reading the manuscript.

Conflicts of Interest: Y.M. (Yoshiaki Minakata) received lecture fees from Nippon Boehringer Ingelheim. The other authors declare no conflicts of interest.

References

1. Lozano, R.; Naghavi, M.; Foreman, K.; Lim, S.; Shibuya, K.; Aboyans, V.; Abraham, J.; Adair, T.; Aggarwal, R.; Ahn, S.Y.; et al. Global and regional mortality from 235 causes of death for 20 age groups in 1990 and 2010: A systematic analysis for the Global Burden of Disease Study 2010. *Lancet* **2012**, *380*, 2095–2128. [CrossRef]
2. Vos, T.; Flaxman, A.D.; Naghavi, M.; Lozano, R.; Michaud, C.; Ezzati, M.; Shibuya, K.; Salomon, J.A.; Abdalla, S.; Aboyans, V.; et al. Years lived with disability (YLDs) for 1160 sequelae of 289 diseases and injuries 1990–2010: A systematic analysis for the Global Burden of Disease Study 2010. *Lancet* **2012**, *380*, 2163–2196. [CrossRef] [PubMed]
3. Mathers, C.D.; Loncar, D. Projections of global mortality and burden of disease from 2002 to 2030. *PLoS Med.* **2006**, *3*, e442. [CrossRef]
4. Pitta, F.; Troosters, T.; Spruit, M.A.; Probst, V.S.; Decramer, M.; Gosselink, R. Characteristics of physical activities in daily life in chronic obstructive pulmonary disease. *Am. J. Respir. Crit. Care Med.* **2005**, *171*, 972–977. [CrossRef]
5. Minakata, Y.; Sugino, A.; Kanda, M.; Ichikawa, T.; Akamatsu, K.; Koarai, A.; Hirano, T.; Nakanishi, M.; Sugiura, H.; Matsunaga, K.; et al. Reduced level of physical activity in Japanese patients with chronic obstructive pulmonary disease. *Respir. Investig.* **2014**, *52*, 41–48. [CrossRef]
6. Jakes, R.W.; Day, N.E.; Patel, B.; Khaw, K.T.; Oakes, S.; Luben, R.; Welch, A.; Bingham, S.; Wareham, N.J. Physical inactivity is associated with lower forced expiratory volume in 1 second: European Prospective Investigation into Cancer-Norfolk Prospective Population Study. *Am. J. Epidemiol.* **2002**, *156*, 139–147. [CrossRef]
7. Pelkonen, M.; Notkola, I.L.; Lakka, T.; Tukiainen, H.O.; Kivinen, P.; Nissinen, A. Delaying decline in pulmonary function with physical activity: A 25-year follow-up. *Am. J. Respir. Crit. Care Med.* **2003**, *168*, 494–499. [CrossRef] [PubMed]
8. Cheng, Y.J.; Macera, C.A.; Addy, C.L.; Sy, F.S.; Wieland, D.; Blair, S.N. Effects of physical activity on exercise tests and respiratory function. *Br. J. Sport. Med.* **2003**, *37*, 521–528. [CrossRef] [PubMed]
9. Garcia-Aymerich, J.; Lange, P.; Benet, M.; Schnohr, P.; Anto, J.M. Regular physical activity modifies smoking-related lung function decline and reduces risk of chronic obstructive pulmonary disease: A population-based cohort study. *Am. J. Respir. Crit. Care Med.* **2007**, *175*, 458–463. [CrossRef]
10. Garcia-Aymerich, J.; Lange, P.; Serra, I.; Schnohr, P.; Antó, J.M. Time-dependent confounding in the study of the effects of regular physical activity in chronic obstructive pulmonary disease: An application of the marginal structural model. *Ann. Epidemiol.* **2008**, *18*, 775–783. [CrossRef]
11. Garcia-Rio, F.; Rojo, B.; Casitas, R.; Lores, V.; Madero, R.; Romero, D.; Galera, R.; Villasante, C. Prognostic value of the objective measurement of daily physical activity in patients with COPD. *Chest* **2012**, *142*, 338–346. [CrossRef]
12. Moy, M.L.; Teylan, M.; Weston, N.A.; Gagnon, D.R.; Garshick, E. Daily Step Count Predicts Acute Exacerbations in a US Cohort with COPD. *PLoS ONE* **2013**, *8*, e60400. [CrossRef]
13. Crook, S.; Busching, G.; Keusch, S.; Wieser, S.; Turk, A.; Frey, M.; Puhan, M.A.; Frei, A. The association between daily exacerbation symptoms and physical activity in patients with chronic obstructive pulmonary disease. *Int. J. Chron. Obs. Pulmon. Dis.* **2018**, *13*, 2199–2206. [CrossRef]
14. Alahmari, A.D.; Patel, A.R.C.; Kowlessar, B.S.; Mackay, A.J.; Singh, R.; Wedzicha, J.A.; Donaldson, G.C. Daily activity during stability and exacerbation of chronic obstructive pulmonary disease. *BMC Pulm. Med.* **2014**, *14*, 98. [CrossRef] [PubMed]
15. Demeyer, H.; Costilla-Frias, M.; Louvaris, Z.; Gimeno-Santos, E.; Tabberer, M.; Rabinovich, R.A.; de Jong, C.; Polkey, M.I.; Hopkinson, N.S.; Karlsson, N.; et al. Both moderate and severe exacerbations accelerate physical activity decline in COPD patients. *Eur. Respir. J.* **2018**, *51*, 1702110. [CrossRef]
16. Garcia-Aymerich, J.; Lange, P.; Benet, M.; Schnohr, P.; Anto, J.M. Regular physical activity reduces hospital admission and mortality in chronic obstructive pulmonary disease: A population based cohort study. *Thorax* **2006**, *61*, 772–778. [CrossRef]
17. Waschki, B.; Kirsten, A.; Holz, O.; Muller, K.C.; Meyer, T.; Watz, H.; Magnussen, H. Physical activity is the strongest predictor of all-cause mortality in patients with COPD: A prospective cohort study. *Chest* **2011**, *140*, 331–342. [CrossRef] [PubMed]
18. Minakata, Y.; Sasaki, S. Data Reproducibility and Effectiveness of Bronchodilators for Improving Physical Activity in COPD Patients. *J. Clin. Med.* **2020**, *9*, 3497. [CrossRef]
19. Caspersen, C.J.; Powell, K.E.; Christenson, G.M. Physical activity, exercise, and physical fitness: Definitions and distinctions for health-related research. *Public Health Rep.* **1985**, *100*, 126–131.
20. Tremblay, M.S.; Colley, R.C.; Saunders, T.J.; Healy, G.N.; Owen, N. Physiological and health implications of a sedentary lifestyle. *Appl. Physiol. Nutr. Metab.* **2010**, *35*, 725–740. [CrossRef] [PubMed]
21. Tremblay, M.S.; Aubert, S.; Barnes, J.D.; Saunders, T.J.; Carson, V.; Latimer-Cheung, A.E.; Chastin, S.F.M.; Altenburg, T.M.; Chinapaw, M.J.M. Sedentary Behavior Research Network (SBRN)—Terminology Consensus Project process and outcome. *Int. J. Behav. Nutr. Phys. Act.* **2017**, *14*, 75. [CrossRef] [PubMed]
22. Lee, I.M.; Shiroma, E.J.; Lobelo, F.; Puska, P.; Blair, S.N.; Katzmarzyk, P.T. Effect of physical inactivity on major non-communicable diseases worldwide: An analysis of burden of disease and life expectancy. *Lancet* **2012**, *380*, 219–229. [CrossRef]

23. Pate, R.R.; O'Neill, J.R.; Lobelo, F. The evolving definition of "sedentary". *Exerc. Sport Sci. Rev.* **2008**, *36*, 173–178. [CrossRef]
24. Network, S.B.R. Letter to the editor: Standardized use of the terms "sedentary" and "sedentary behaviours". *Appl. Physiol. Nutr. Metab.* **2012**, *37*, 540–542.
25. Furlanetto, K.C.; Donaria, L.; Schneider, L.P.; Lopes, J.R.; Ribeiro, M.; Fernandes, K.B.; Hernandes, N.A.; Pitta, F. Sedentary Behavior Is an Independent Predictor of Mortality in Subjects with COPD. *Respir. Care* **2017**, *62*, 579–587. [CrossRef] [PubMed]
26. Ukawa, S.; Tamakoshi, A.; Yatsuya, H.; Yamagishi, K.; Ando, M.; Iso, H. Association between Average Daily Television Viewing Time and Chronic Obstructive Pulmonary Disease-Related Mortality: Findings from the Japan Collaborative Cohort Study. *J. Epidemiol.* **2015**, *25*, 431–436. [CrossRef]
27. Cavalheri, V.; Straker, L.; Gucciardi, D.F.; Gardiner, P.A.; Hill, K. Changing physical activity and sedentary behaviour in people with COPD. *Respirology* **2016**, *21*, 419–426. [CrossRef] [PubMed]
28. Lewis, L.K.; Hunt, T.; Williams, M.T.; English, C.; Olds, T.S. Sedentary Behavior in People with and without a Chronic Health Condition: How Much, What and When? *AIMS Public Health* **2016**, *3*, 503–519. [CrossRef]
29. McKeough, Z.; Cheng, S.W.M.; Alison, J.; Jenkins, C.; Hamer, M.; Stamatakis, E. Low leisure-based sitting time and being physically active were associated with reduced odds of death and diabetes in people with chronic obstructive pulmonary disease: A cohort study. *J. Physiother.* **2018**, *64*, 114–120. [CrossRef] [PubMed]
30. Dogra, S.; Good, J.; Buman, M.P.; Gardiner, P.A.; Copeland, J.L.; Stickland, M.K. Physical activity and sedentary time are related to clinically relevant health outcomes among adults with obstructive lung disease. *BMC Pulm. Med.* **2018**, *18*, 98. [CrossRef]
31. Bernard, P.; Hains-Monfette, G.; Atoui, S.; Moullec, G. Daily Objective Physical Activity and Sedentary Time in Adults with COPD Using Spirometry Data from Canadian Measures Health Survey. *Can. Respir. J.* **2018**, *2018*, 9107435. [CrossRef] [PubMed]
32. Ichinose, M.; Minakata, Y.; Motegi, T.; Takahashi, T.; Seki, M.; Sugaya, S.; Hayashi, N.; Kuwahira, I. A Non-Interventional, Cross-Sectional Study to Evaluate Factors Relating to Daily Step Counts and Physical Activity in Japanese Patients with Chronic Obstructive Pulmonary Disease: STEP COPD. *Int. J. Chron. Obs. Pulmon. Dis.* **2020**, *15*, 3385–3396. [CrossRef] [PubMed]
33. Sievi, N.A.; Brack, T.; Brutsche, M.H.; Frey, M.; Irani, S.; Leuppi, J.D.; Thurnheer, R.; Kohler, M.; Clarenbach, C.F. Accelerometer- versus questionnaire-based assessment of physical activity and their changes over time in patients with COPD. *Int. J. Chron. Obs. Pulmon. Dis.* **2017**, *12*, 1113–1118. [CrossRef]
34. Thyregod, M.; Bodtger, U. Coherence between self-reported and objectively measured physical activity in patients with chronic obstructive lung disease: A systematic review. *Int. J. Chron. Obs. Pulmon. Dis.* **2016**, *11*, 2931–2938. [CrossRef]
35. Van Remoortel, H.; Raste, Y.; Louvaris, Z.; Giavedoni, S.; Burtin, C.; Langer, D.; Wilson, F.; Rabinovich, R.; Vogiatzis, I.; Hopkinson, N.S.; et al. Validity of six activity monitors in chronic obstructive pulmonary disease: A comparison with indirect calorimetry. *PLoS ONE* **2012**, *7*, e39198. [CrossRef]
36. de Groot, S.; Nieuwenhuizen, M.G. Validity and reliability of measuring activities, movement intensity and energy expenditure with the DynaPort MoveMonitor. *Med. Eng. Phys.* **2013**, *35*, 1499–1505. [CrossRef]
37. Rabinovich, R.A.; Louvaris, Z.; Raste, Y.; Langer, D.; Van Remoortel, H.; Giavedoni, S.; Burtin, C.; Regueiro, E.M.; Vogiatzis, I.; Hopkinson, N.S.; et al. Validity of physical activity monitors during daily life in patients with COPD. *Eur. Respir. J.* **2013**, *42*, 1205–1215. [CrossRef]
38. Farooqi, N.; Slinde, F.; Håglin, L.; Sandström, T. Validation of SenseWear Armband and ActiHeart monitors for assessments of daily energy expenditure in free-living women with chronic obstructive pulmonary disease. *Physiol. Rep.* **2013**, *1*, e00150. [CrossRef] [PubMed]
39. Steele, B.G.; Holt, L.; Belza, B.; Ferris, S.; Lakshminaryan, S.; Buchner, D.M. Quantitating physical activity in COPD using a triaxial accelerometer. *Chest* **2000**, *117*, 1359–1367. [CrossRef]
40. Hunt, T.; Williams, M.T.; Olds, T.S. Reliability and validity of the multimedia activity recall in children and adults (MARCA) in people with chronic obstructive pulmonary disease. *PLoS ONE* **2013**, *8*, e81274. [CrossRef] [PubMed]
41. Sugino, A.; Minakata, Y.; Kanda, M.; Akamatsu, K.; Koarai, A.; Hirano, T.; Sugiura, H.; Matsunaga, K.; Ichinose, M. Validation of a compact motion sensor for the measurement of physical activity in patients with chronic obstructive pulmonary disease. *Respiration* **2012**, *83*, 300–307. [CrossRef] [PubMed]
42. Miyamoto, S.; Minakata, Y.; Azuma, Y.; Kawabe, K.; Ono, H.; Yanagimoto, R.; Suruda, T. Verification of a Motion Sensor for Evaluating Physical Activity in COPD Patients. *Can. Respir. J.* **2018**, *2018*, 8343705. [CrossRef]
43. Turner, L.J.; Houchen, L.; Williams, J.; Singh, S.J. Reliability of pedometers to measure step counts in patients with chronic respiratory disease. *J. Cardiopulm. Rehabil. Prev.* **2012**, *32*, 284–291. [CrossRef] [PubMed]
44. Hartmann, A.; Luzi, S.; Murer, K.; de Bie, R.A.; de Bruin, E.D. Concurrent validity of a trunk tri-axial accelerometer system for gait analysis in older adults. *Gait Posture* **2009**, *29*, 444–448. [CrossRef]
45. Harrison, S.L.; Horton, E.J.; Smith, R.; Sandland, C.J.; Steiner, M.C.; Morgan, M.D.; Singh, S.J. Physical activity monitoring: Addressing the difficulties of accurately detecting slow walking speeds. *Heart Lung* **2013**, *42*, 361–364.e1. [CrossRef]
46. Feng, Y.; Wong, C.K.; Janeja, V.; Kuber, R.; Mentis, H.M. Comparison of tri-axial accelerometers step-count accuracy in slow walking conditions. *Gait Posture* **2017**, *53*, 11–16. [CrossRef]
47. Oshima, Y.; Kawaguchi, K.; Tanaka, S.; Ohkawara, K.; Hikihara, Y.; Ishikawa-Takata, K.; Tabata, I. Classifying household and locomotive activities using a triaxial accelerometer. *Gait Posture* **2010**, *31*, 370–374. [CrossRef]

48. Ohkawara, K.; Oshima, Y.; Hikihara, Y.; Ishikawa-Takata, K.; Tabata, I.; Tanaka, S. Real-time estimation of daily physical activity intensity by a triaxial accelerometer and a gravity-removal classification algorithm. *Br. J. Nutr.* **2011**, *105*, 1681–1691. [CrossRef] [PubMed]
49. Alahmari, A.D.; Mackay, A.J.; Patel, A.R.; Kowlessar, B.S.; Singh, R.; Brill, S.E.; Allinson, J.P.; Wedzicha, J.A.; Donaldson, G.C. Influence of weather and atmospheric pollution on physical activity in patients with COPD. *Respir. Res.* **2015**, *16*, 71. [CrossRef]
50. Balish, S.M.; Dechman, G.; Hernandez, P.; Spence, J.C.; Rhodes, R.E.; McGannon, K.; Blanchard, C. The Relationship between Weather and Objectively Measured Physical Activity among Individuals with COPD. *J. Cardiopulm. Rehabil. Prev.* **2017**, *37*, 445–449. [CrossRef]
51. Vaidya, T.; Thomas-Ollivier, V.; Hug, F.; Bernady, A.; Le Blanc, C.; de Bisschop, C.; Chambellan, A. Translation and Cultural Adaptation of PROactive Instruments for COPD in French and Influence of Weather and Pollution on Its Difficulty Score. *Int. J. Chron. Obs. Pulmon. Dis.* **2020**, *15*, 471–478. [CrossRef]
52. Sumukadas, D.; Witham, M.; Struthers, A.; McMurdo, M. Day length and weather conditions profoundly affect physical activity levels in older functionally impaired people. *J. Epidemiol. Community Health* **2009**, *63*, 305–309. [CrossRef] [PubMed]
53. Sewell, L.; Singh, S.J.; Williams, J.E.; Morgan, M.D. Seasonal variations affect physical activity and pulmonary rehabilitation outcomes. *J. Cardiopulm. Rehabil. Prev.* **2010**, *30*, 329–333. [CrossRef]
54. Furlanetto, K.C.; Demeyer, H.; Sant'anna, T.; Hernandes, N.A.; Camillo, C.A.; Pons, I.S.; Gosselink, R.; Troosters, T.; Pitta, F. Physical Activity of Patients with COPD from Regions with Different Climatic Variations. *COPD* **2017**, *14*, 276–283. [CrossRef]
55. Donaldson, G.C.; Goldring, J.J.; Wedzicha, J.A. Influence of season on exacerbation characteristics in patients with COPD. *Chest* **2012**, *141*, 94–100. [CrossRef]
56. Gretebeck, R.J.; Montoye, H.J. Variability of some objective measures of physical activity. *Med. Sci. Sport. Exerc.* **1992**, *24*, 1167–1172. [CrossRef]
57. Matthews, C.E.; Ainsworth, B.E.; Thompson, R.W.; Bassett, D.R., Jr. Sources of variance in daily physical activity levels as measured by an accelerometer. *Med. Sci. Sport. Exerc.* **2002**, *34*, 1376–1381. [CrossRef] [PubMed]
58. Tudor-Locke, C.; Burkett, L.; Reis, J.P.; Ainsworth, B.E.; Macera, C.A.; Wilson, D.K. How many days of pedometer monitoring predict weekly physical activity in adults? *Prev Med.* **2005**, *40*, 293–298. [CrossRef]
59. Troiano, R.P.; Berrigan, D.; Dodd, K.W.; Masse, L.C.; Tilert, T.; McDowell, M. Physical activity in the United States measured by accelerometer. *Med. Sci. Sport. Exerc.* **2008**, *40*, 181–188. [CrossRef]
60. Choi, L.; Liu, Z.; Matthews, C.E.; Buchowski, M.S. Validation of accelerometer wear and nonwear time classification algorithm. *Med. Sci. Sport. Exerc.* **2011**, *43*, 357–364. [CrossRef] [PubMed]
61. Choi, L.; Ward, S.C.; Schnelle, J.F.; Buchowski, M.S. Assessment of wear/nonwear time classification algorithms for triaxial accelerometer. *Med. Sci. Sport. Exerc.* **2012**, *44*, 2009–2016. [CrossRef] [PubMed]
62. Byrom, B.; Rowe, D.A. Measuring free-living physical activity in COPD patients: Deriving methodology standards for clinical trials through a review of research studies. *Contemp. Clin. Trials* **2016**, *47*, 172–184. [CrossRef] [PubMed]
63. Demeyer, H.; Burtin, C.; Van Remoortel, H.; Hornikx, M.; Langer, D.; Decramer, M.; Gosselink, R.; Janssens, W.; Troosters, T. Standardizing the analysis of physical activity in patients with COPD following a pulmonary rehabilitation program. *Chest* **2014**, *146*, 318–327. [CrossRef] [PubMed]
64. Kantorowski, A.; Wan, E.S.; Homsy, D.; Kadri, R.; Richardson, C.R.; Moy, M.L. Determinants and outcomes of change in physical activity in COPD. *ERJ Open Res.* **2018**, *4*, 00054-2018. [CrossRef] [PubMed]
65. Hains-Monfette, G.; Atoui, S.; Needham Dancause, K.; Bernard, P. Device-Assessed Physical Activity and Sedentary Behaviors in Canadians with Chronic Disease(s): Findings from the Canadian Health Measures Survey. *Sports* **2019**, *7*, 113. [CrossRef]
66. Minakata, Y.; Motegi, T.; Ueki, J.; Gon, Y.; Nakamura, S.; Anzai, T.; Hirata, K.; Ichinose, M. Effect of tiotropium/olodaterol on sedentary and active time in patients with COPD: Post hoc analysis of the VESUTO((R)) study. *Int. J. Chron. Obs. Pulmon. Dis.* **2019**, *14*, 1789–1801. [CrossRef]
67. Hoaas, H.; Zanaboni, P.; Hjalmarsen, A.; Morseth, B.; Dinesen, B.; Burge, A.T.; Cox, N.S.; Holland, A.E. Seasonal variations in objectively assessed physical activity among people with COPD in two Nordic countries and Australia: A cross-sectional study. *Int. J. Chron. Obs. Pulmon. Dis.* **2019**, *14*, 1219–1228. [CrossRef]
68. Paneroni, M.; Ambrosino, N.; Simonelli, C.; Bertacchini, L.; Venturelli, M.; Vitacca, M. Physical Activity in Patients with Chronic Obstructive Pulmonary Disease on Long-Term Oxygen Therapy: A Cross-Sectional Study. *Int. J. Chron. Obs. Pulmon. Dis.* **2019**, *14*, 2815–2823. [CrossRef]
69. Watz, H.; Waschki, B.; Meyer, T.; Magnussen, H. Physical activity in patients with COPD. *Eur. Respir. J.* **2009**, *33*, 262–272. [CrossRef]
70. Nakanishi, M.; Minakata, Y.; Tanaka, R.; Sugiura, H.; Kuroda, H.; Yoshida, M.; Yamamoto, N. Simple standard equation for daily step count in Japanese patients with chronic obstructive pulmonary disease. *Int. J. Chron. Obs. Pulmon. Dis.* **2019**, *14*, 1967–1977. [CrossRef]
71. Minakata, Y.; Sasaki, S.; Azuma, Y.; Kawabe, K.; Ono, H. Reference Equations for Assessing the Physical Activity of Japanese Patients with Chronic Obstructive Pulmonary Disease. *Int. J. Chron. Obs. Pulmon. Dis.* **2021**, *16*, 3041–3053. [CrossRef]
72. Waschki, B.; Spruit, M.A.; Watz, H.; Albert, P.S.; Shrikrishna, D.; Groenen, M.; Smith, C.; Man, W.D.; Tal-Singer, R.; Edwards, L.D.; et al. Physical activity monitoring in COPD: Compliance and associations with clinical characteristics in a multicenter study. *Respir. Med.* **2012**, *106*, 522–530. [CrossRef] [PubMed]

73. Van Remoortel, H.; Hornikx, M.; Demeyer, H.; Langer, D.; Burtin, C.; Decramer, M.; Gosselink, R.; Janssens, W.; Troosters, T. Daily physical activity in subjects with newly diagnosed COPD. *Thorax* **2013**, *68*, 962–963. [CrossRef]
74. Demeyer, H.; Gimeno-Santos, E.; Rabinovich, R.A.; Hornikx, M.; Louvaris, Z.; de Boer, W.I.; Karlsson, N.; de Jong, C.; Van der Molen, T.; Vogiatzis, I.; et al. Physical Activity Characteristics across GOLD Quadrants Depend on the Questionnaire Used. *PLoS ONE* **2016**, *11*, e0151255. [CrossRef] [PubMed]
75. Okubadejo, A.A.; O'Shea, L.; Jones, P.W.; Wedzicha, J.A. Home assessment of activities of daily living in patients with severe chronic obstructive pulmonary disease on long-term oxygen therapy. *Eur. Respir. J.* **1997**, *10*, 1572–1575. [CrossRef]
76. Lahaije, A.J.; van Helvoort, H.A.; Dekhuijzen, P.N.; Vercoulen, J.H.; Heijdra, Y.F. Resting and ADL-induced dynamic hyperinflation explain physical inactivity in COPD better than FEV1. *Respir. Med.* **2013**, *107*, 834–840. [CrossRef]
77. Shiue, I. Daily walking > 10 min could improve mental health in people with historical cardiovascular disease or COPD: Scottish Health Survey, 2012. *Int. J. Cardiol.* **2015**, *179*, 375–377. [CrossRef] [PubMed]
78. Arbillaga-Etxarri, A.; Gimeno-Santos, E.; Barberan-Garcia, A.; Benet, M.; Borrell, E.; Dadvand, P.; Foraster, M.; Marin, A.; Monteagudo, M.; Rodriguez-Roisin, R.; et al. Socio-environmental correlates of physical activity in patients with chronic obstructive pulmonary disease (COPD). *Thorax* **2017**, *72*, 796–802. [CrossRef]
79. Tanimura, K.; Sato, S.; Fuseya, Y.; Hasegawa, K.; Uemasu, K.; Sato, A.; Oguma, T.; Hirai, T.; Mishima, M.; Muro, S. Quantitative Assessment of Erector Spinae Muscles in Patients with Chronic Obstructive Pulmonary Disease. *Nov. Chest Comput. Tomogr.-Deriv. Index Prognosis. Ann. Am. Thorac. Soc.* **2016**, *13*, 334–341.
80. Shrikrishna, D.; Patel, M.; Tanner, R.J.; Seymour, J.M.; Connolly, B.A.; Puthucheary, Z.A.; Walsh, S.L.; Bloch, S.A.; Sidhu, P.S.; Hart, N.; et al. Quadriceps wasting and physical inactivity in patients with COPD. *Eur. Respir. J.* **2012**, *40*, 1115–1122. [CrossRef] [PubMed]
81. Ijiri, N.; Kanazawa, H.; Asai, K.; Watanabe, T.; Hirata, K. Irisin, a newly discovered myokine, is a novel biomarker associated with physical activity in patients with chronic obstructive pulmonary disease. *Respirology* **2015**, *20*, 612–617. [CrossRef]
82. Tanaka, R.; Sugiura, H.; Yamada, M.; Ichikawa, T.; Koarai, A.; Fujino, N.; Yanagisawa, S.; Onodera, K.; Numakura, T.; Sato, K.; et al. Physical inactivity is associated with decreased growth differentiation factor 11 in chronic obstructive pulmonary disease. *Int. J. Chron. Obs. Pulmon. Dis.* **2018**, *13*, 1333–1342. [CrossRef]
83. Moy, M.L.; Teylan, M.; Weston, N.A.; Gagnon, D.R.; Danilack, V.A.; Garshick, E. Daily step count is associated with plasma C-reactive protein and IL-6 in a US cohort with COPD. *Chest* **2014**, *145*, 542–550. [CrossRef] [PubMed]
84. Fischer, C.P.; Berntsen, A.; Perstrup, L.B.; Eskildsen, P.; Pedersen, B.K. Plasma levels of interleukin-6 and C-reactive protein are associated with physical inactivity independent of obesity. *Scand. J. Med. Sci. Sport.* **2007**, *17*, 580–587. [CrossRef]
85. Fuertes, E.; Carsin, A.E.; Garcia-Larsen, V.; Guerra, S.; Pin, I.; Leynaert, B.; Accordini, S.; Martinez-Moratalla, J.; Anto, J.M.; Urrutia, I.; et al. The role of C-reactive protein levels on the association of physical activity with lung function in adults. *PLoS ONE* **2019**, *14*, e0222578. [CrossRef] [PubMed]
86. Taka, C.; Hayashi, R.; Shimokawa, K.; Tokui, K.; Okazawa, S.; Kambara, K.; Inomata, M.; Yamada, T.; Matsui, S.; Tobe, K. SIRT1 and FOXO1 mRNA expression in PBMC correlates to physical activity in COPD patients. *Int. J. Chron. Obs. Pulmon. Dis.* **2017**, *12*, 3237–3244. [CrossRef] [PubMed]
87. Burge, A.T.; Cox, N.S.; Abramson, M.J.; Holland, A.E. Interventions for promoting physical activity in people with chronic obstructive pulmonary disease (COPD). *Cochrane Database Syst. Rev.* **2020**, *4*, Cd012626. [CrossRef]
88. Hataji, O.; Naito, M.; Ito, K.; Watanabe, F.; Gabazza, E.C.; Taguchi, O. Indacaterol improves daily physical activity in patients with chronic obstructive pulmonary disease. *Int. J. Chron. Obs. Pulmon. Dis.* **2013**, *8*, 1–5.
89. Watz, H.; Krippner, F.; Kirsten, A.; Magnussen, H.; Vogelmeier, C. Indacaterol improves lung hyperinflation and physical activity in patients with moderate chronic obstructive pulmonary disease–a randomized, multicenter, double-blind, placebo-controlled study. *BMC Pulm. Med.* **2014**, *14*, 158. [CrossRef]
90. Minakata, Y.; Morishita, Y.; Ichikawa, T.; Akamatsu, K.; Hirano, T.; Nakanishi, M.; Matsunaga, K.; Ichinose, M. Effects of pharmacologic treatment based on airflow limitation and breathlessness on daily physical activity in patients with chronic obstructive pulmonary disease. *Int. J. Chron. Obs. Pulmon. Dis.* **2015**, *10*, 1275–1282. [CrossRef]
91. Watz, H.; Troosters, T.; Beeh, K.M.; Garcia-Aymerich, J.; Paggiaro, P.; Molins, E.; Notari, M.; Zapata, A.; Jarreta, D.; Garcia Gil, E. ACTIVATE: The effect of aclidinium/formoterol on hyperinflation, exercise capacity, and physical activity in patients with COPD. *Int. J. Chron. Obs. Pulmon. Dis.* **2017**, *12*, 2545–2558. [CrossRef] [PubMed]
92. Kamei, T.; Nakamura, H.D.; Nanki, N.D.; Minakata, Y.D.; Matsunaga, K.D.; Mori, Y.D. Clinical benefit of two-times-per-day aclidinium bromide compared with once-a-day tiotropium bromide hydrate in COPD: A multicentre, open-label, randomised study. *BMJ Open* **2019**, *9*, e024114. [CrossRef]
93. Hirano, T.; Matsunaga, K.; Hamada, K.; Uehara, S.; Suetake, R.; Yamaji, Y.; Oishi, K.; Asami, M.; Edakuni, N.; Ogawa, H.; et al. Combination of assist use of short-acting beta-2 agonists inhalation and guidance based on patient-specific restrictions in daily behavior: Impact on physical activity of Japanese patients with chronic obstructive pulmonary disease. *Respir. Investig.* **2019**, *57*, 133–139. [CrossRef]
94. Tsujimura, Y.; Hiramatsu, T.; Kojima, E.; Tabira, K. Effect of pulmonary rehabilitation with assistive use of short-acting β2 agonist in COPD patients using long-acting bronchodilators. *Physiother. Theory Pract.* **2019**, *37*, 719–728. [CrossRef] [PubMed]

95. Beeh, K.M.; Watz, H.; Puente-Maestu, L.; de Teresa, L.; Jarreta, D.; Caracta, C.; Gil, E.G.; Magnussen, H. Aclidinium improves exercise endurance, dyspnea, lung hyperinflation, and physical activity in patients with COPD: A randomized, placebo-controlled, crossover trial. *BMC Pulm. Med.* **2014**, *14*, 209. [CrossRef]
96. Nishijima, Y.; Minami, S.; Yamamoto, S.; Ogata, Y.; Koba, T.; Futami, S.; Komuta, K. Influence of indacaterol on daily physical activity in patients with untreated chronic obstructive pulmonary disease. *Int. J. Chron. Obs. Pulmon. Dis.* **2015**, *10*, 439–444.
97. Watz, H.; Mailander, C.; Baier, M.; Kirsten, A. Effects of indacaterol/glycopyrronium (QVA149) on lung hyperinflation and physical activity in patients with moderate to severe COPD: A randomised, placebo-controlled, crossover study (The MOVE Study). *BMC Pulm. Med.* **2016**, *16*, 95. [CrossRef] [PubMed]
98. O'Donnell, D.E.; Casaburi, R.; Vincken, W.; Puente-Maestu, L.; Swales, J.; Lawrence, D.; Kramer, B. Effect of indacaterol on exercise endurance and lung hyperinflation in COPD. *Respir. Med.* **2011**, *105*, 1030–1036. [CrossRef] [PubMed]
99. Troosters, T.; Sciurba, F.C.; Decramer, M.; Siafakas, N.M.; Klioze, S.S.; Sutradhar, S.C.; Weisman, I.M.; Yunis, C. Tiotropium in patients with moderate COPD naive to maintenance therapy: A randomised placebo-controlled trial. *NPJ Prim. Care Respir. Med.* **2014**, *24*, 14003. [CrossRef] [PubMed]
100. Ichinose, M.; Minakata, Y.; Motegi, T.; Ueki, J.; Gon, Y.; Seki, T.; Anzai, T.; Nakamura, S.; Hirata, K. Efficacy of tiotropium/olodaterol on lung volume, exercise capacity, and physical activity. *Int. J. Chron. Obs. Pulmon. Dis.* **2018**, *13*, 1407–1419. [CrossRef]
101. Troosters, T.; Maltais, F.; Leidy, N.; Lavoie, K.L.; Sedeno, M.; Janssens, W.; Garcia-Aymerich, J.; Erzen, D.; De Sousa, D.; Korducki, L.; et al. Effect of Bronchodilation, Exercise Training, and Behavior Modification on Symptoms and Physical Activity in Chronic Obstructive Pulmonary Disease. *Am. J. Respir. Crit. Care Med.* **2018**, *198*, 1021–1032. [CrossRef]
102. Miravitlles, M.; García-Rivero, J.L.; Ribera, X.; Galera, J.; García, A.; Palomino, R.; Pomares, X. Exercise capacity and physical activity in COPD patients treated with a LAMA/LABA combination: A systematic review and meta-analysis. *Respir. Res.* **2022**, *23*, 347. [CrossRef]
103. Shioya, T.; Sato, S.; Iwakura, M.; Takahashi, H.; Terui, Y.; Uemura, S.; Satake, M. Improvement of physical activity in chronic obstructive pulmonary disease by pulmonary rehabilitation and pharmacological treatment. *Respir. Investig.* **2018**, *56*, 292–306. [CrossRef]
104. Locke, E.A.; Latham, G.P. *A Theory of Goal Setting & Task Performance*; Prentice-Hall, Inc.: Englewood Cliffs, NJ, USA, 1990.
105. Altenburg, W.A.; ten Hacken, N.H.; Bossenbroek, L.; Kerstjens, H.A.; de Greef, M.H.; Wempe, J.B. Short- and long-term effects of a physical activity counselling programme in COPD: A randomised controlled trial. *Respir. Med.* **2015**, *109*, 112–121. [CrossRef] [PubMed]
106. Moy, M.L.; Collins, R.J.; Martinez, C.H.; Kadri, R.; Roman, P.; Holleman, R.G.; Kim, H.M.; Nguyen, H.Q.; Cohen, M.D.; Goodrich, D.E.; et al. An Internet-Mediated Pedometer-Based Program Improves Health-Related Quality-of-Life Domains and Daily Step Counts in COPD: A Randomized Controlled Trial. *Chest* **2015**, *148*, 128–137. [CrossRef]
107. Wan, E.S.; Kantorowski, A.; Homsy, D.; Teylan, M.; Kadri, R.; Richardson, C.R.; Gagnon, D.R.; Garshick, E.; Moy, M.L. Promoting physical activity in COPD: Insights from a randomized trial of a web-based intervention and pedometer use. *Respir. Med.* **2017**, *130*, 102–110. [CrossRef]
108. Moy, M.L.; Martinez, C.H.; Kadri, R.; Roman, P.; Holleman, R.G.; Kim, H.M.; Nguyen, H.Q.; Cohen, M.D.; Goodrich, D.E.; Giardino, N.D.; et al. Long-Term Effects of an Internet-Mediated Pedometer-Based Walking Program for Chronic Obstructive Pulmonary Disease: Randomized Controlled Trial. *J. Med. Internet Res.* **2016**, *18*, e215. [CrossRef] [PubMed]
109. Robinson, S.A.; Wan, E.S.; Shimada, S.L.; Richardson, C.R.; Moy, M.L. Age and Attitudes Towards an Internet-Mediated, Pedometer-Based Physical Activity Intervention for Chronic Obstructive Pulmonary Disease: Secondary Analysis. *JMIR Aging* **2020**, *3*, e19527. [CrossRef] [PubMed]
110. Sasaki, S.; Minakata, Y.; Azuma, Y.; Kaki, T.; Kawabe, K.; Ono, H. Effects of individualized target setting on step count in Japanese patients with chronic obstructive pulmonary disease: A pilot study. *Adv. Respir. Med.* **2022**, *90*, 1–8. [CrossRef]
111. Owen, N.; Healy, G.N.; Matthews, C.E.; Dunstan, D.W. Too much sitting: The population health science of sedentary behavior. *Exerc. Sport Sci. Rev.* **2010**, *38*, 105–113. [CrossRef]
112. Biswas, A.; Oh, P.I.; Faulkner, G.E.; Bajaj, R.R.; Silver, M.A.; Mitchell, M.S.; Alter, D.A. Sedentary time and its association with risk for disease incidence, mortality, and hospitalization in adults: A systematic review and meta-analysis. *Ann. Intern. Med.* **2015**, *162*, 123–132. [CrossRef]
113. Loprinzi, P.D.; Lee, H.; Cardinal, B.J. Evidence to support including lifestyle light-intensity recommendations in physical activity guidelines for older adults. *Am. J. Health Promot.* **2015**, *29*, 277–284. [CrossRef] [PubMed]
114. Ekelund, U.; Tarp, J.; Steene-Johannessen, J.; Hansen, B.H.; Jefferis, B.; Fagerland, M.W.; Whincup, P.; Diaz, K.M.; Hooker, S.P.; Chernofsky, A.; et al. Dose-response associations between accelerometry measured physical activity and sedentary time and all cause mortality: Systematic review and harmonised meta-analysis. *BMJ* **2019**, *366*, l4570. [CrossRef] [PubMed]
115. Piercy, K.L.; Troiano, R.P.; Ballard, R.M.; Carlson, S.A.; Fulton, J.E.; Galuska, D.A.; George, S.M.; Olson, R.D. The Physical Activity Guidelines for Americans. *JAMA* **2018**, *320*, 2020–2028. [CrossRef]
116. Diaz, K.M.; Duran, A.T.; Colabianchi, N.; Judd, S.E.; Howard, V.J.; Hooker, S.P. Potential Effects on Mortality of Replacing Sedentary Time with Short Sedentary Bouts or Physical Activity: A National Cohort Study. *Am. J. Epidemiol.* **2019**, *188*, 537–544. [CrossRef]

117. Katzmarzyk, P.T.; Church, T.S.; Craig, C.L.; Bouchard, C. Sitting time and mortality from all causes, cardiovascular disease, and cancer. *Med. Sci. Sport. Exerc.* **2009**, *41*, 998–1005. [CrossRef]
118. Grontved, A.; Hu, F.B. Television viewing and risk of type 2 diabetes, cardiovascular disease, and all-cause mortality: A meta-analysis. *JAMA* **2011**, *305*, 2448–2455. [CrossRef]
119. Young, D.R.; Hivert, M.F.; Alhassan, S.; Camhi, S.M.; Ferguson, J.F.; Katzmarzyk, P.T.; Lewis, C.E.; Owen, N.; Perry, C.K.; Siddique, J.; et al. Sedentary Behavior and Cardiovascular Morbidity and Mortality: A Science Advisory from the American Heart Association. *Circulation* **2016**, *134*, e262–e279. [CrossRef] [PubMed]
120. Dunstan, D.W.; Howard, B.; Healy, G.N.; Owen, N. Too much sitting—A health hazard. *Diabetes Res. Clin. Pract.* **2012**, *97*, 368–376. [CrossRef]
121. Colberg, S.R.; Sigal, R.J.; Yardley, J.E.; Riddell, M.C.; Dunstan, D.W.; Dempsey, P.C.; Horton, E.S.; Castorino, K.; Tate, D.F. Physical Activity/Exercise and Diabetes: A Position Statement of the American Diabetes Association. *Diabetes Care* **2016**, *39*, 2065–2079. [CrossRef]
122. Vineis, P.; Wild, C.P. Global cancer patterns: Causes and prevention. *Lancet* **2014**, *383*, 549–557. [CrossRef] [PubMed]
123. Patterson, R.; McNamara, E.; Tainio, M.; de Sá, T.H.; Smith, A.D.; Sharp, S.J.; Edwards, P.; Woodcock, J.; Brage, S.; Wijndaele, K. Sedentary behaviour and risk of all-cause, cardiovascular and cancer mortality, and incident type 2 diabetes: A systematic review and dose response meta-analysis. *Eur. J. Epidemiol.* **2018**, *33*, 811–829. [CrossRef] [PubMed]
124. Patel, A.V.; Friedenreich, C.M.; Moore, S.C.; Hayes, S.C.; Silver, J.K.; Campbell, K.L.; Winters-Stone, K.; Gerber, L.H.; George, S.M.; Fulton, J.E.; et al. American College of Sports Medicine Roundtable Report on Physical Activity, Sedentary Behavior, and Cancer Prevention and Control. *Med. Sci. Sport. Exerc.* **2019**, *51*, 2391–2402. [CrossRef] [PubMed]
125. Chan, D.S.M.; Abar, L.; Cariolou, M.; Nanu, N.; Greenwood, D.C.; Bandera, E.V.; McTiernan, A.; Norat, T. World Cancer Research Fund International: Continuous Update Project-systematic literature review and meta-analysis of observational cohort studies on physical activity, sedentary behavior, adiposity, and weight change and breast cancer risk. *Cancer Causes Control* **2019**, *30*, 1183–1200. [CrossRef]
126. Dempsey, P.C.; Owen, N.; Biddle, S.J.; Dunstan, D.W. Managing sedentary behavior to reduce the risk of diabetes and cardiovascular disease. *Curr. Diabetes Rep.* **2014**, *14*, 522. [CrossRef] [PubMed]
127. Azuma, Y.; Minakata, Y.; Kaki, T.; Sasaki, S.; Kawabe, K.; Ono, H. Time spent by COPD patients lying down during sedentary behavior. *Health Educ. Public Health* **2021**, *4*, 415–420.
128. Takahashi, K.; Uchida, M.; Kato, G.; Takamori, A.; Kinoshita, T.; Yoshida, M.; Tajiri, R.; Kojima, K.; Inoue, H.; Kobayashi, H.; et al. First-Line Treatment with Tiotropium/Olodaterol Improves Physical Activity in Patients with Treatment-Naïve Chronic Obstructive Pulmonary Disease. *Int. J. Chron. Obs. Pulmon. Dis.* **2020**, *15*, 2115–2126. [CrossRef] [PubMed]
129. Orme, M.; Weedon, A.; Esliger, D.; Saukko, P.; Morgan, M.; Steiner, M.; Downey, J.; Singh, S.; Sherar, L. Study protocol for Chronic Obstructive Pulmonary Disease-Sitting and ExacerbAtions Trial (COPD-SEAT): A randomised controlled feasibility trial of a home-based self-monitoring sedentary behaviour intervention. *BMJ Open* **2016**, *6*, e013014. [CrossRef]
130. Geidl, W.; Carl, J.; Cassar, S.; Lehbert, N.; Mino, E.; Wittmann, M.; Wagner, R.; Schultz, K.; Pfeifer, K. Physical Activity and Sedentary Behaviour Patterns in 326 Persons with COPD before Starting a Pulmonary Rehabilitation: A Cluster Analysis. *J. Clin. Med.* **2019**, *8*, 1346. [CrossRef]
131. Wootton, S.L.; Hill, K.; Alison, J.A.; Ng, L.W.C.; Jenkins, S.; Eastwood, P.R.; Hillman, D.R.; Jenkins, C.; Spencer, L.; Cecins, N.; et al. Effects of ground-based walking training on daily physical activity in people with COPD: A randomised controlled trial. *Respir. Med.* **2017**, *132*, 139–145. [CrossRef] [PubMed]
132. Mesquita, R.; Meijer, K.; Pitta, F.; Azcuna, H.; Goertz, Y.M.J.; Essers, J.M.N.; Wouters, E.F.M.; Spruit, M.A. Changes in physical activity and sedentary behaviour following pulmonary rehabilitation in patients with COPD. *Respir. Med.* **2017**, *126*, 122–129. [CrossRef] [PubMed]
133. Orme, M.W.; Steiner, M.C.; Morgan, M.D.; Kingsnorth, A.P.; Esliger, D.W.; Singh, S.J.; Sherar, L.B. 24-hour accelerometry in COPD: Exploring physical activity, sedentary behavior, sleep and clinical characteristics. *Int. J. Chron. Obs. Pulmon. Dis.* **2019**, *14*, 419–430. [CrossRef] [PubMed]
134. Cheng, S.W.M.; Alison, J.; Stamatakis, E.; Dennis, S.; McNamara, R.; Spencer, L.; McKeough, Z. Six-week behaviour change intervention to reduce sedentary behaviour in people with chronic obstructive pulmonary disease: A randomised controlled trial. *Thorax* **2022**, *77*, 231–238. [CrossRef] [PubMed]
135. Takahashi, K.; Tashiro, H.; Tajiri, R.; Takamori, A.; Uchida, M.; Kato, G.; Kurihara, Y.; Sadamatsu, H.; Kinoshita, T.; Yoshida, M.; et al. Factors Associated with Reduction of Sedentary Time Following Tiotropium/Olodaterol Therapy in Treatment-Naïve Chronic Obstructive Pulmonary Disease. *Int. J. Chron. Obs. Pulmon. Dis.* **2021**, *16*, 3297–3307. [CrossRef] [PubMed]

Disclaimer/Publisher's Note: The statements, opinions and data contained in all publications are solely those of the individual author(s) and contributor(s) and not of MDPI and/or the editor(s). MDPI and/or the editor(s) disclaim responsibility for any injury to people or property resulting from any ideas, methods, instructions or products referred to in the content.

Article

Physical Activity Estimated by the Wearable Device in Lung Disease Patients: Exploratory Analyses of Prospective Observational Study

Kentaro Ito [1,2,*], Maki Esumi [1], Seiya Esumi [1], Yuta Suzuki [1], Tadashi Sakaguchi [1], Kentaro Fujiwara [1], Yoichi Nishii [1], Hiroki Yasui [1], Osamu Taguchi [1] and Osamu Hataji [1]

1. Respiratory Center, Matsusaka Municipal Hospital, Matsusaka 515-0073, Japan
2. Biostatistics, Yokohama City University, Yokohama 236-0004, Japan
* Correspondence: kentarou_i_0214@yahoo.co.jp

Abstract: Background. Physical activity is a potential parameter to assess the severity or prognosis of lung disease. However, the differences in physical activity between healthy individuals and patients with lung disease remain unclear. **Methods.** The analyses in this report are a combined analysis of four cohorts, including a healthy control cohort, in a prospective study designed to evaluate wearable device-estimated physical activity in three cohorts: the lung cancer cohort, the interstitial pneumonia cohort, and the COPD cohort (UMIN000047834). In this report, physical activity in the lung disease cohort was compared with that in the healthy cohort. Subgroup analyses were performed based on age, sex, duration of wearable device use, and lung disease subtype. **Results.** A total of 238 cases were analyzed, including 216 patients with lung disease and 22 healthy cases. Distance walked and number of steps were significantly lower in the patient group compared to the healthy control group. ROC analysis for the diagnostic value of lung disease by mean distance walked and mean number of steps showed AUC of 0.764 (95%CI, 0.673 to 0.856) and 0.822 (95%CI, 0.740 to 0.905), respectively. There was a significant difference in physical activity by age, but not by gender nor by duration based on the threshold of 7 days of wearing the device. **Conclusions.** Lung disease decreases physical activity compared to healthy subjects, and aging may bias the estimation of physical activity. The distance walked or number of steps is recommended as a measure of physical activity, with a period of approximately one week and adjusted for age for future investigation.

Keywords: physical activity; lung disease/pulmonary disease; healthy case; wearable fitness tracker device

1. Introduction

Physical activity is an important parameter to evaluate an individual's general health status. Some reports have indicated the importance of physical activity in patients with lung diseases, especially COPD [1–5]. reports about the difference in physical activity between the patients with lung diseases and healthy cases were limited. In practice, there are even some patients with serious diseases, such as lung cancer, who show full activity that is not inferior to that of healthy individuals. Therefore, we investigated whether there is a difference in physical activity between patients and healthy individuals before discussing whether the measurement of physical activity is available to assess the severity of a specific disease. We hypothesized that there is difference in physical activity between the healthy population and lung disease population and that the physical activity value is available for evaluating the general status among lung disease population. The aim of this exploratory analysis is to investigating the hypothesis. We first identified the useful measurements with a comparison of each physical activity between the healthy population and lung disease population, and investigate the diagnostic value of physical activity for lung disease. We expected that METS and distance walked would correlate better with disease status and prognosis than step count, so we used a wearable device that could measure all of these. The data of the three cohorts and healthy control in a prospective study to evaluate disease severity by physical activity estimated by wearable device were used for the analyses as an exploratory investigation.

2. Materials and Methods

2.1. Patients

The results of this report are from exploratory analysis of the main study, which was designed to assess disease severity in three disease cohorts using a wearable device (UMIN000047834), and the aim of this analysis was to compare physical activity between healthy cases and patients with lung disease.

The main study is a prospective observational study at a single-institution, and the inclusion criteria included (1) patients diagnosed with advanced lung cancer, interstitial pneumonia or COPD, and (2) outpatients for treatment or observation at a single institution. Patients with interstitial pneumonia were enrolled regardless of the type of interstitial pneumonia, from interstitial pulmonary fibrosis to collagen-disease-related interstitial pneumonia, and patients with COPD were diagnosed in clinical practice based on pulmonary function testing. The exclusion criteria included (1) patients with unstable gait due to lower limb disease. Healthy controls without lung disease were recruited from the medical staff. The healthy group was enrolled as an exploratory group, separate from the other three cohorts in this analysis, for the purpose of exploratory validation as an exploratory study group.

2.2. Measurement of Physical Activity

We used the wearable device, amue link (SONY, Inc., Tokyo, Japan), which is equipped with a GPS system that can monitor real time movements without any other device, such as smart phone. To estimate the distance walked, this device adopts a unique algorithm to distinguish the method of travel, such as by vehicle or on foot. This device is also expected to calculate the actual walked distance. In this study, this device measured a total of 6 physical activity values as follows: sum and mean of (1) METS, (2) distance walked, and (3) number of steps. All patients were instructed to wear the wearable device on their wrist, following the company's recommendation that the device on the wrist can adequately measure distance walked and steps taken. The duration of measurement was from wake-up to bedtime, with the exception of special situations such as bath time. All participants were instructed to wear the fitness tracker device for up to 14 days. The data were sent to the data center via the Internet and stored in real time with the reservation of privacy.

2.3. Outcome

The wearable device measurements were compared between the healthy and lung disease groups, and we estimated the AUC to discriminate the healthy from lung disease groups by physical activity in the ROC analysis. Although the aim was not to discriminate disease by physical activity, we assumed that the high accuracy of discriminating disease by physical activity, represented by a higher AUC, means that physical activity is associated with the presence or absence of respiratory disease. Comparisons of physical activity were made between patients with lung disease and healthy controls, and between the different types of lung disease. We hypothesized that the factors of age, sex, and the duration the device is worn may bias the estimation of physical activity and subgroup analyses performed based on these factors.

2.4. Statistics and Ethics

As described above, physical activity, as continuous values, were compared between patients with lung disease and healthy controls, and between different types of lung disease. The physical activity values were compared between the healthy group and lung disease using the Kruskal–Wallis test, and the multiple comparison tests across groups were performed using the Dunn–Bonferroni method. Statistical comparisons of the continuous values were tested with 0.05 representing a significant difference. ROC analyses were performed, and the 95% confidential intervals were calculated by SPSS version 28.0. As this is an exploratory study, sample size calculations were not performed. We obtained written informed consent from all enrolled cases and followed them prospectively in this study. The study was conducted in accordance with the principles of the Declaration of Helsinki.

3. Results

3.1. Characteristics

A total of 238 cases were analyzed, including 22 healthy cases, 119 patients with lung cancer, 51 patients with interstitial pneumonia, and 46 patients with COPD (Table 1). Written informed consent was obtained from all enrolled cases, and we observed them prospectively. For all cases, the median age was 73 years (range, 24 to 88) and the duration of device wear was 8 days. The median and the duration of wear were not significantly different in each group, but the age is significantly younger in the healthy group compared to the other groups ($p < 0.001$). The failure rate for physical activity assessment in the whole population is 5.5%. The physical activities measured by the wearable device showed a stronger correlation with each other, except for METS.

Table 1. Characteristics.

	All	Healthy Control	Pulmonary Disease	Lung Cancer	Interstitial Pneumonia	COPD
N	238	22	216	119	51	46
Median age [range]	73 (24–88)	36 (24–58)	74 (32–88)	72 (32–88)	74 (54–85)	75 (43–83)
≥75 years old	99 (41.6%)	0 (0%)	99 (45.8%)	47 (39.5%)	24 (47.1%)	28 (60.9%)
Sex M/F	152/86	9/13	143/73	71/48	34/17	38/8
Wearing days, median	8	9	7	7	8	7
≤7 days	117 (49.2%)	7 (31.8%)	110 (50.9%)	60 (50.4%)	25 (49.0%)	25 (54.3%)
Failure to estimate PA	13 (5.5%)	0 (0%)	13 (%)	8 (6.7%)	0 (0%)	5 (10.9%)

Abbreviation: Physical activity, PA; Chronic obstruct pulmonary disease, COPD.

3.2. Healthy vs. Pulmonary Disease

Nonparametric test was performed for the measured value estimated by the wearable device between groups. As a result, the distance walked and the number of steps walked were candidate parameters as physical activities for diagnosis of lung disease. The physical activities in the patient group were statistically significantly lower compared with the healthy control group, with p value of 0.05 or less for the sum of METS, sum and mean of the distance walked, and sum and mean of the number of steps walked (Figure 1). ROC analysis for the diagnostic value of lung disease by distance walked showed an AUC of 0.764 (95%CI, 0.673 to 0.856) (Figure 2).

3.3. Across the Subtype of Pulmonary Disease

There was significant difference in physical activity in except with METS between healthy control group and each lung disease group (Table 2). For all lung diseases, the physical activity has trend to be decreased compared with healthy control group, and the largest difference compared with healthy group was found in lung cancer cohort, while the smallest difference was in COPD cohort (Figure 3).

3.4. Subgroups by Age, Gender, and the Wearing Period

Subgroup analysis by age showed that patients aged 75 years or older had less physical activity in all disease subtypes, and distance and steps walked were significantly different between younger and older patients (Figure 4). There was no difference in physical activity between men and women in all disease subtypes, except for COPD, where the sample size of women was very small. Analyses based on time worn showed that there was no difference in physical activity between 7 or fewer days worn and 8 or more days worn. This trend is consistent across lung disease subtypes, so the data suggest that one week may be a sufficient estimation period. Finally, based on these results, we hypothesized that age may be biased in discriminating the reason for lower physical activity due to disease status or aging. Therefore, we conducted an ROC analysis in the subgroup of 69 or younger cases, which resulted in an AUC of 0.732 (95%CI, 0.617 to 0.848) to 0.825 (95%CI, 0.721 to 0.929) (Figure 5).

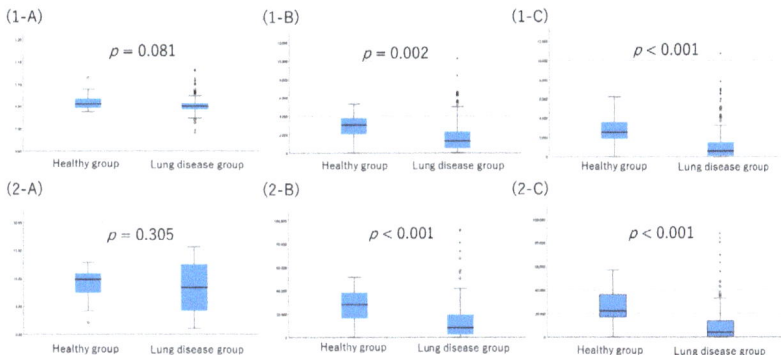

Figure 1. Comparison of physical activity estimated by ePRO between healthy group and pulmonary disease group. Three parameters of physical activity were shown as (**1-A,2-A**) METS, (**1-B,2-B**) distance walked, and (**1-C,2-C**) number of steps of (**1-A–1-C**) the average (on the top) and (**2-A–2-C**) the total (on the bottom). In a box plot, the box represents the interquartile range, with its top and bottom indicating the third and first quartiles, respectively. The whiskers extend from the box to cover the data within an area 1.5 times the size of the interquartile range. Data points outside this range are considered outliers and are represented as dots.

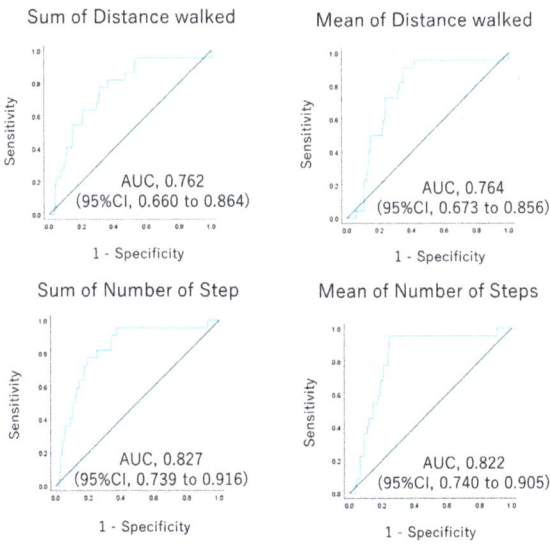

Figure 2. AUC for diagnosis with lung disease by physical activity in ROC analysis. Blue line is ROC curves of sum of distance walked or mean of distance walked. Green line is a reference line.

Table 2. Kruskal–Wallis test and multiple comparison test by Dunn-Bonferroni method for each paired groups.

Parameter of Physical Activity to Subtype of Pulmonary Disease for Null Hypothesis	Kruskal–Wallis Test	Multiple Comparison Test					
		LK vs. IP	LK vs. CO	LK vs. HE	IP vs. CO	IP vs. HE	CO vs. HE
Sum of METS	0.769						
Mean of METS	0.090						
Sum of distance walked	<0.001	0.892	0.596	<0.001	0.723	<0.001	0.002
Mean of distance walked	<0.001	0.842	0.178	<0.001	0.310	<0.001	0.006
Sum of steps walked	<0.001	0.609	0.437	<0.001	0.276	<0.001	<0.001
Mean of steps walked	<0.001	0.409	0.219	<0.001	0.083	<0.001	<0.001

Abbreviations: LK, lung cancer; CO, COPD; IP, interstitial pneumonia; HE, healthy control case.

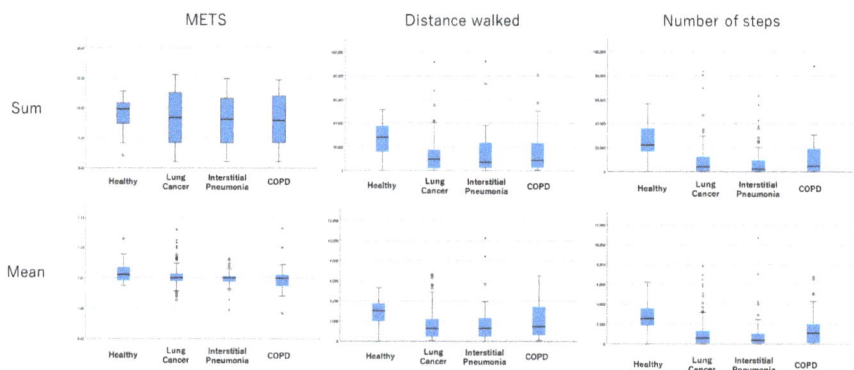

Figure 3. Physical activity in each lung disease subtype. In each graph, from left to right, healthy cases, lung cancer patients, interstitial pneumonia patients, and COPD patients. In a box plot, the box represents the interquartile range, with its top and bottom indicating the third and first quartiles, respectively. The whiskers extend from the box to cover the data within an area 1.5 times the size of the interquartile range. Data points outside this range are considered outliers and are represented as dots.

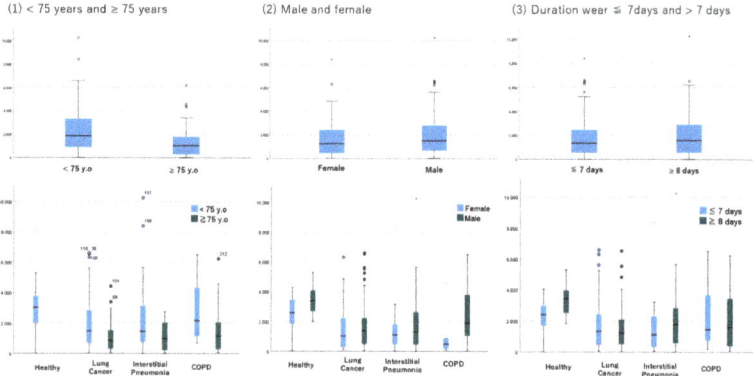

Figure 4. Subgroup analyses based on age, sex, and the duration worn. Comparison of mean distance walked between (**left**) <75 years and ≥75 years, (**middle**) female and male, (**right**) worn less than 7 days and more than 7 days. Each comparison based on lung disease is shown in the bottom row. In a box plot, the box represents the interquartile range, with its top and bottom indicating the third and first quartiles, respectively. The whiskers extend from the box to cover the data within an area 1.5 times the size of the interquartile range. Data points outside this range are considered outliers and are represented as dots.

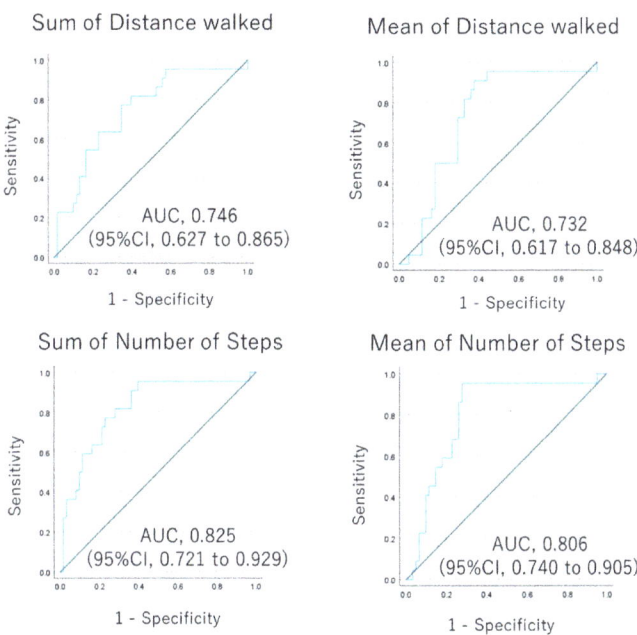

Figure 5. ROC analysis for diagnosis with pulmonary disease in the subgroup of cases with age less than 70. Blue line is ROC curves of sum of distance walked or mean of distance walked. Green line is a reference line.

4. Discussion

The analyses in this study indicated the following three important clinical questions: (1) which measurement among wearable device is appropriate to assess physical activity, (2) which factor should be adjusted, and (3) how long of a term is required to estimate physical activity?

Our data showed a significant difference in physical activity between the patients with lung disease and healthy cases. In previous reports, Fabio Pitta et al. reported that patients with COPD were inactive compared with healthy elderly patients [6], and Benoit Wallaert et al. reported that the patients with fibrotic idiopathic interstitial pneumonia also had less activity in their daily lives compared to healthy controls [7], which is consistent with the results of our study. However, there was a significant difference in age between these two groups, which was further investigated in the subgroup analyses.

A greater difference was found in the lung cancer group followed by interstitial pneumonia group among three cohort, from which we expect that an measurement of physical activity will be of clinical significance, especially in the two pulmonary diseases. Sofie Breuls et al. showed that the patients with interstitial pneumonia were less active compared with the patients with COPD in their propensity score analysis. This study used the daily steps to evaluate the physical activity [8]. As we can see in Figure 3, our data also showed that the physical activity, in both distance walked and steps walked, were lower in the interstitial pneumonia group compared with the COPD group. In addition, the proportion of the patients aged 75 or older was higher in the COPD group, with 47.1% in the interstitial pneumonia group and 60.9% in the COPD group, which supports the inactivity of patients with interstitial pneumonia.

There was a significant difference in the distance walked and the number of steps walked between each disease cohort and the healthy group, and these two measurements seemed to be the candidate parameters of physical activities in our study. In our study, METS is not a better candidate to evaluate the physical activity, however, the formula for estimating METS is specified for the device, therefore, the results in our study do not mean that METS is not completely excluded as a parameter of physical activity when using the other device. The previous study, as mentioned above, assessed physical activity using steps, and our data also showed that the number of steps walked was a better predictor of lower physical activity due to lung disease. Meanwhile, our data showed that mean distance walked also had potential as a candidate measure of physical activity in the lung disease population. In particular, this device, amue link, was designed to calculate the distance by using a unique algorithm to identify movement on foot, which may be the reason why the distance walked was a better predictor of physical activity in this study.

The subgroup analyses based on age, sex, or duration of device wear showed that age may be a bias for physical activity, suggesting that these measured activities require adjustment based on age but not sex. Therefore, we performed an additional subgroup analysis of cases of individuals aged 69 or younger, in which the difference in physical activity between patients and healthy controls has remained consistent, and the AUC in this subgroup is 0.732 (95%CI, 0.617 to 0.848), which is not as inferior compared to that in all cases (0.764 (95%CI, 0.673 to 0.856)). The decrease in physical activity with age has been reported in the previous reports [9–11], which is consistent with our results. However, the female sex has also been reported to be associated with a decreased physical activity [10], which was not confirmed in our study, probably because of the imbalance in the proportion of male and female participants. This indicates that a decreased physical activity is not only due to aging, but also to lung disease, so the assessment of physical activity in patients with lung disease should be performed in any disease cohort with adjustment for age. The subgroup based on the days of wearing the device showed that the duration of physical activity estimation may be sufficient to be approximately one week. However, the results were suggestive rather than conclusive, and further confirmation is needed for them to be associated with disease severity, even after adjusting for age.

This study has some limitations. Failure to measure physical activity was calculated to occur at 5.5%, which may bias the analysis. There are some outliers in the data, which are assumed to be caused by errors with the device in estimating physical activity. The analyses were not prospectively designed, and the sample size of the healthy control group is small, although the sample size of the pulmonary disease group is sufficiently large, which may be a limitation. In addition, it is inevitable that the variation across disease will be a limitation of the analysis.

5. Conclusions

The lung disease decreased the physical activity compared with healthy cases in our study. Considering the fact that the difference in physical activity between healthy case and lung disease patients, the physical activity had potential to be reflected on the severity of the disease. We are preparing to report the association between the lung disease severity and physical activity in the next report of this study, which is the primary endpoint of the main study. Our data showed that age should be adjusted for when assessing physical activity, but the reduced physical activity in patients with lung disease was found even in the younger population. The subtype of lung disease seems to be associated with reduced physical activity. The number of steps walked was a good parameter of physical activity in our study, as shown in the previous study indicated. In addition, the distance walked was also a good indicator of daily activity when calculated by the device used in our study. We recommend using the distance or steps walked as a measure of physical activity with the period of about one week while adjusting for age for future investigations.

Author Contributions: Conceptualization, K.I. and O.H.; methodology, K.I.; validation, K.I., O.H. and O.T.; formal analysis, K.I.; investigation, K.I., M.E., S.E., Y.S., T.S., K.F., Y.N., H.Y., O.T. and O.H.; resources, K.I.; data curation, K.I.; writing—original draft preparation, K.I.; writing—review and editing, O.H., O.T. and H.Y.; visualization, K.I.; supervision, O.T.; project administration, K.I. All authors have read and agreed to the published version of the manuscript.

Funding: This research received no external funding.

Institutional Review Board Statement: The study was conducted in accordance with the Declaration of Helsinki and approved by the Institutional Review Board of Matsusaka Municipal Hospital (approval number: 210604-5-3, date: 4 June 2021).

Informed Consent Statement: Informed consent was obtained from all subjects involved in the study.

Data Availability Statement: The data in this study will be available in accordance with Japanese law for personal privacy protection by request to the corresponding author.

Acknowledgments: We thank the patients, patients' families, investigators, and medical staff who supported this study.

Conflicts of Interest: The authors declare no conflict of interest.

References

1. Liao, S.Y.; Benzo, R.; Ries, A.L.; Soler, X. Physical Activity Monitoring in Patients with Chronic Obstructive Pulmonary Disease. *Chronic Obstr. Pulm. Dis.* **2014**, *1*, 155–165. [CrossRef] [PubMed]
2. Esteban, C.; Quintana, J.M.; Aburto, M.; Moraza, J.; Egurrola, M.; Pérez-Izquierdo, J.; Aizpiri, S.; Aguirre, U.; Capelastegui, A. Impact of changes in physical activity on health-related quality of life among patients with COPD. *Eur. Respir. J.* **2010**, *36*, 292–300. [CrossRef] [PubMed]
3. Garcia-Aymerich, J.; Lange, P.; Benet, M.; Schnohr, P.; Antó, J.M. Regular physical activity reduces hospital admission and mortality in chronic obstructive pulmonary disease: A population based cohort study. *Thorax* **2006**, *61*, 772–778. [CrossRef] [PubMed]
4. Dhillon, H.M.; Bell, M.L.; van der Ploeg, H.P.; Turner, J.D.; Kabourakis, M.; Spencer, L.; Lewis, C.; Hui, R.; Blinman, P.; Clarke, S.J.; et al. Impact of physical activity on fatigue and quality of life in people with advanced lung cancer: A randomized controlled trial. *Ann. Oncol.* **2017**, *28*, 1889–1897. [CrossRef] [PubMed]
5. Nakayama, M.; Bando, M.; Araki, K.; Sekine, T.; Kurosaki, F.; Sawata, T.; Nakazawa, S.; Mato, N.; Yamasawa, H.; Sugiyama, Y. Physical activity in patients with idiopathic pulmonary fibrosis. *Respirology* **2015**, *20*, 640–646. [CrossRef] [PubMed]
6. Pitta, F.; Troosters, T.; Spruit, M.A.; Probst, V.S.; Decramer, M.; Gosselink, R. Characteristics of physical activities in daily life in chronic obstructive pulmonary disease. *Am. J. Respir. Crit. Care Med.* **2005**, *171*, 972–977. [CrossRef]
7. Wallaert, B.; Monge, E.; Le Rouzic, O.; Wémeau-Stervinou, L.; Salleron, J.; Grosbois, J.M. Physical activity in daily life of patients with fibrotic idiopathic interstitial pneumonia. *Chest* **2013**, *144*, 1652–1658. [CrossRef]
8. Breuls, S.; Pereira de Araujo, C.; Blondeel, A.; Yserbyt, J.; Janssens, W.; Wuyts, W.; Troosters, T.; Demeyer, H. Physical activity pattern of patients with interstitial lung disease compared to patients with COPD: A propensity-matched study. *PLoS ONE* **2022**, *17*, e0277973. [CrossRef]
9. Ishikawa-Takata, K.; Nakae, S.; Sasaki, S.; Katsukawa, F.; Tanaka, S. Age-Related Decline in Physical Activity Level in the Healthy Older Japanese Population. *J. Nutr. Sci. Vitaminol.* **2021**, *67*, 330–338. [CrossRef]
10. da Silva, I.C.; van Hees, V.T.; Ramires, V.V.; Knuth, A.G.; Bielemann, R.M.; Ekelund, U.; Brage, S.; Hallal, P.C. Physical activity levels in three Brazilian birth cohorts as assessed with raw triaxial wrist accelerometry. *Int. J. Epidemiol.* **2014**, *43*, 1959–1968. [CrossRef]
11. Mielke, G.I.; Burton, N.W.; Brown, W.J. Accelerometer-measured physical activity in mid-age Australian adults. *BMC Public Health* **2022**, *22*, 1952. [CrossRef]

Disclaimer/Publisher's Note: The statements, opinions and data contained in all publications are solely those of the individual author(s) and contributor(s) and not of MDPI and/or the editor(s). MDPI and/or the editor(s) disclaim responsibility for any injury to people or property resulting from any ideas, methods, instructions or products referred to in the content.

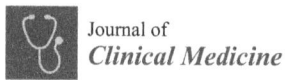

Article

Neural Network Approach to Investigating the Importance of Test Items for Predicting Physical Activity in Chronic Obstructive Pulmonary Disease

Yoshiki Nakahara [1], Shingo Mabu [1,*], Tsunahiko Hirano [2], Yoriyuki Murata [2], Keiko Doi [2], Ayumi Fukatsu-Chikumoto [2] and Kazuto Matsunaga [2]

[1] Graduate School of Sciences and Technology for Innovation, Yamaguchi University, Yamaguchi 7558611, Japan
[2] Department of Respiratory Medicine and Infectious Disease, Yamaguchi University Hospital, Yamaguchi 7558505, Japan
* Correspondence: mabu@yamaguchi-u.ac.jp

Abstract: Contracting COPD reduces a patient's physical activity and restricts everyday activities (physical activity disorder). However, the fundamental cause of physical activity disorder has not been found. In addition, costly and specialized equipment is required to accurately examine the disorder; hence, it is not regularly assessed in normal clinical practice. In this study, we constructed a machine learning model to predict physical activity using test items collected during the normal care of COPD patients. In detail, we first applied three types of data preprocessing methods (zero-padding, multiple imputation by chained equations (MICE), and k-nearest neighbor (kNN)) to complement missing values in the dataset. Then, we constructed several types of neural networks to predict physical activity. Finally, permutation importance was calculated to identify the importance of the test items for prediction. Multifactorial analysis using machine learning, including blood, lung function, walking, and chest imaging tests, was the unique point of this research. From the experimental results, it was found that the missing value processing using MICE contributed to the best prediction accuracy (73.00%) compared to that using zero-padding (68.44%) or kNN (71.52%), and showed better accuracy than XGBoost (66.12%) with a significant difference ($p < 0.05$). For patients with severe physical activity reduction (total exercise < 1.5), a high sensitivity (89.36%) was obtained. The permutation importance showed that "sex, the number of cigarettes, age, and the whole body phase angle (nutritional status)" were the most important items for this prediction. Furthermore, we found that a smaller number of test items could be used in ordinary clinical practice for the screening of physical activity disorder.

Keywords: COPD; physical activity; prediction; neural network; autoencoder

1. Introduction

Chronic obstructive pulmonary disease (COPD) is a chronic inflammatory disease of the lungs that is primarily caused by smoking, which causes the occlusion of airflow and prevents the return to normal function according to respiration function tests [1]. Airflow limitation and air trapping lead to the static and dynamic hyperinflation of the lungs. In turn, this causes patients to have difficulty breathing during laborious tasks, leading to a reduction in exercise tolerance and physical activity as measured by the indicators of activity time and the amount of physical activity at each level of exercise intensity. This is called physical activity disorder. In other words, if COPD patients suffer from reductions in their exercise ability, this leads to reduced physical activity, which in turn leads to a vicious cycle of reduced muscle strength and worse prognosis [2–5]. In addition, COPD patients may not be aware of their respiratory symptoms because they are physically inactive, i.e., some patients are physically inactive even though they feel few respiratory symptoms.

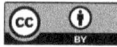

This suggests that it is difficult to make immediate judgements regarding actual physical activity in clinical settings. Physical activity is regulated by various factors, which can make physical activity disorder challenging to understand and assess in patients with COPD. However, the mechanism of physical activity disorder that worsens COPD and appropriate treatment targets have not been found. In addition, there are many related test items and running all possible tests incurs significant costs. As a result, in the treatment of COPD, it is important to find relevant test items to predict physical activity with high accuracy.

Previous research on predicting physical activity has included predictions made with and without machine learning. As an example of predictions using machine learning, pulse rate data were used to predict the physical activity of elderly patients [6]. In [7], the physical activity of children not yet in preschool was predicted using a random forest method. In [8], data provided by sensor chips capable of being adapted for use in mobility assistance devices, such as canes or crutches, were used to make predictions using machine learning. In [9], accelerometer bracelets were used to predict physical activity using various machine learning models. In [10], physical activity was predicted using experimental processes of change (experimental POCs), behavioral processes of change (behavioral POCs), and interactions between the two. Research using deep learning has also been conducted, including a proposed physical activity prediction model that used long short-term memory recurrent neural networks [11]. In [12], factors associated with low-intensity physical activity were examined using multivariate regression analysis. In [13], the effectiveness of a simple prediction equation for step counts obtained using multivariate regression analysis was evaluated by comparing the predicted values to actual measured values. Some research has been conducted without using machine learning, including [14], which investigated whether it was possible to predict domain-specific physical activity 20 years later in adulthood using domain-specific physical activity in early childhood. Similarly, Ref. [15] investigated the extent to which adult physical activity patterns could be predicted using physical characteristics, physical abilities, and activity levels during adolescence. In [16], physical activity and metabolic equivalents (METs) per day were predicted using three commercially available accelerometers and eight regression equations. Ref. [17] applied the Fogg behavior model and the transtheoretical behavior model to predict physical activity. In [18], the authors examined the association between physical activity and the expiratory to inspiratory (E/I) ratio of mean lung density (MLD) and showed that the E/I ratio of MLD could be a useful imaging biomarker for the early detection of physical inactivity in COPD patients.

On the other hand, machine learning models for predicting the physical activity of COPD patients using multifactorial test data, including blood, lung function, walking, and chest imaging tests, have not been constructed. Therefore, in this study, we attempted to build a typical neural network model for physical activity prediction using various types of test items and evaluated its prediction performance. Generally, in machine learning, a large amount of training data is required. However, since collecting a sufficient amount of data for specific diseases from one medical institution is difficult, the proposed prediction model applied pre-training using an autoencoder [19]. Since physical activity is defined by a variety of factors, it is difficult to predict physical activity disorder using simple tests in ordinary clinical practice. Therefore, the main aims of this study were as follows: (1) to clarify whether physical activity could be predicted using machine learning and measure the prediction performance; (2) to clarify which test items were important for prediction using a method called permutation importance; (3) to examine the applicability of machine learning for the diagnosis of physical activity disorder through (1) and (2), even in local hospitals with access to only simple tests.

2. Materials and Methods

2.1. Ethics Approval and Consent to Participate

This study was approved by the Institutional Review Board of Yamaguchi University Hospital (H27-204) and was conducted according to the principles of the Declaration of Helsinki. Informed consent was obtained from all individuals included in this study.

2.2. Dataset

The dataset used in this study was composed of 406 cases of patient data provided by the Department of Respiratory Medicine and Infectious Disease, Yamaguchi University Hospital, Japan (COPD patients, non-COPD patients, and healthy individuals). The non-COPD patients were patients with respiratory illnesses other than COPD, such as bronchial asthma, bronchiectasis, and interstitial pneumonia. The numbers of patients in each category were 143 COPD patients, 238 non-COPD patients, and 25 healthy individuals. Data were collected for 32 test items, including questionnaires regarding respiratory symptoms, whole body phase angle, blood tests, lung function tests, and computed tomography (CT) images. The activity monitor we used (produced by Omron) measured and aggregated exercise (Ex) from the number of steps and activity levels during each hour from 0:00 to 23:00. Ex was computed by multiplying activity intensity (METs) by time, and only exercise with an intensity of 3.0 METs or more was used to calculate Ex. Physical activity represents the performance of physical actions, so smaller values indicated reductions in physical activity. Total exercise (T-Ex) values of less than 3 (METs × hr) were defined as abnormal physical activity, while those of 3 (METs × hr) or more were considered normal physical activity, as previously reported in [20]. Based on the above data, we trained a neural network to classify each patient as displaying either normal or abnormal physical activity. The explanatory variables were the 32 test items (the inputs to the neural network) and the response variable was physical activity (i.e., Total Exercise or T-Ex (the output from the neural network)). When applying these data to machine learning, each value was normalized to fall between a minimum of 0 and a maximum of 1. Detailed information about the variables is presented in Table 1. Note that importance index in Table 1 will be explained in later sections. However, as not every test was performed for each patient, the data were missing some values. Thus, one of the three missing value imputation methods (zero-padding, multiple imputation by chained equations (MICE) [21], and k-nearest neighbor (kNN) [22]) was used to complement missing values.

2.3. Missing Value Processing

The outlines of the three missing value processing methods (zero-padding, MICE, and kNN) are as follows:

- Zero-padding just replaces missing values with zeros;
- MICE handles missing values by predicting them (in detail, MICE builds a machine learning model that predicts missing values for certain test items by using the values of the other test items);
- kNN handles missing values by using values of the nearest data from the data with missing values.

Table 1. The basic data statistics for each test item and the statistics of their permutation importance. The test items are sorted by their mean importance. The data statistics for Sex (M/F) show the numbers of males and females. Note: CI, confidence interval; STD, standard deviation; DDR, desaturation distance ratio; mMRC, modified British medical research council; FEV_1, predicted forced expiratory volume in 1s (%); RV, residual volume; TLC, total lung capacity; BNP, brain natriuretic peptide; GDF-15, growth differentiation factor-15; DL_{CO}, diffusing capacity of the lungs for carbon monoxide; VC, vital capacity; VA, alveolar volume; DE/DI, the ratio of mean lung density at the end of expiration (E) to the end of inspiration (I); FeNO, fractional exhaled nitric oxide; LAA, low-attenuation area; ALB, albumin; NDE/NDI, the ratio of normal density at the end of expiration (E) to the end of inspiration (I); DSP, distance–saturation product; CAT, COPD assessment test; BMI, body mass index.

	Data Statistics		Importance Index					
	Mean	STD	Mean	Min	1st Quartile	Median	3rd Quartile	Max	95% CI (Lower–Upper)
Sex (M/F)	309/97		0.051	−0.200	−0.013	0.024	0.100	0.400	−0.013–0.116
# of Cigarettes/Day	16.28	14.10	0.038	−0.100	0.000	0.048	0.051	0.211	0.008–0.068
Age	70.15	9.57	0.035	−0.095	0.000	0.049	0.053	0.190	0.003–0.066
Whole Body Phase Angle (°)	5.07	0.76	0.028	−0.238	0.000	0.048	0.064	0.143	−0.011–0.066
DDR/s	5.91	6.09	0.024	−0.095	0.000	0.000	0.050	0.095	0.003–0.046
mMRC	0.68	0.89	0.023	−0.143	0.000	0.000	0.051	0.190	−0.012–0.058
FEV_1	2.19	0.64	0.017	−0.095	0.000	0.048	0.048	0.105	−0.005–0.040
%RV/TLC (%)	95.52	16.81	0.015	−0.095	0.000	0.000	0.048	0.095	−0.005–0.035
Pack Years	28.17	20.67	0.014	−0.100	0.000	0.000	0.050	0.095	−0.011–0.039
BNP (pg/mL)	38.08	49.48	0.013	−0.050	0.000	0.000	0.050	0.095	−0.007–0.032
GDF-15 (pg/mL)	1245	853	0.008	−0.050	−0.048	0.000	0.048	0.105	−0.017–0.032
Spinal Muscles (Left) (mm²)	1550	436	0.007	−0.053	0.000	0.000	0.000	0.100	−0.008–0.023
DL_{CO}	96.25	27.25	0.007	−0.050	0.000	0.000	0.048	0.053	−0.008–0.023
Grip Strength (Left) (Kg)	29.43	8.51	0.005	−0.100	0.000	0.000	0.048	0.105	−0.018–0.028
Eosinophil	3.63	4.60	0.005	−0.050	0.000	0.000	0.000	0.053	−0.008–0.018
%FEV_1 (%)	85.28	21.28	0.005	−0.050	0.000	0.000	0.012	0.050	−0.010–0.019
VC (L)	3.33	0.81	0.003	−0.050	0.000	0.000	0.000	0.100	−0.013–0.018
%DLCOVA (%)	88.32	38.08	0.002	−0.050	0.000	0.000	0.000	0.050	−0.007–0.011
DE/DI	0.96	0.03	0.002	−0.050	0.000	0.000	0.000	0.095	−0.011–0.016
%VC (%)	99.95	17.04	0.002	−0.050	0.000	0.000	0.000	0.050	−0.009–0.014
FeNO (ppb)	33.70	31.40	0.002	−0.050	0.000	0.000	0.000	0.095	−0.011–0.016
LAA (%)	0.23	0.04	0.000	−0.050	0.000	0.000	0.000	0.050	−0.015–0.015
ALB (g/dL)	4.20	0.31	0.000	−0.050	0.000	0.000	0.000	0.053	−0.013–0.013
NDE/NDI	0.92	0.03	0.000	0.000	0.000	0.000	0.000	0.000	—
FEV_1 (%)	66.62	12.29	−0.000	−0.050	0.000	0.000	0.000	0.050	−0.015–0.015
Spinal Muscles (Right) (mm²)	1586	437	−0.003	−0.050	0.000	0.000	0.000	0.000	−0.008–0.003
DSP	38,082	8404	−0.003	−0.053	0.000	0.000	0.000	0.050	−0.012–0.007
Lowest SpO2 (%)	91.98	3.83	−0.003	−0.050	0.000	0.000	0.000	0.048	−0.012–0.006
6MWT (m)	412.40	85.02	−0.005	−0.053	0.000	0.000	0.000	0.050	−0.015–0.005
Charlson Index	0.96	1.04	−0.006	−0.100	−0.048	0.000	0.000	0.095	−0.032–0.021
CAT	10.87	7.44	−0.007	−0.095	−0.048	0.000	0.012	0.050	−0.027–0.012
BMI (kg/m²)	22.73	3.60	−0.010	−0.200	0.000	0.000	0.000	0.050	−0.037–0.017

The detailed procedures for MICE and kNN are as follows:

- MICE is a multiple imputation method in which missing values are predicted through regression using other feature values. Below, the explanatory variables of the dataset (the values of each of the test items) are referred to as $x_1, x_2, \ldots, x_q$ in the MICE sequence. The explanatory variables are called feature values hereinafter.
    1. An initial value (e.g., mean value) is assigned to each missing value to create pseudo-complete data;
    2. If x_1 is a missing value, x_1 is returned to the missing state and a regression model (e.g., linear regression) is used on the pseudo-complete data $x_2, x_3, \ldots, x_q$ to produce and replace x_1 with the imputed value;
    3. The imputed values for x_2 and onward are generated and replaced, just as in step 2;
    4. The procedure from steps 2–3 is repeated an arbitrary number of times. MICE is a method that updates imputed values sequentially. In this study, the initial values were set as the means of the corresponding features and linear regression was used.

- kNN is a supervised learning classification algorithm. In kNN, the given data are plotted on a feature space and if unknown class data appear, the k points of the data are selected in the order of proximity to the unknown class data and the unknown class data are categorized into classes based on the majority of these k points. Euclidean distance was used to compute distance and $k = 1$, i.e., the k-nearest neighbor algorithm, was used for missing value processing in our preliminary experiments. In kNN with $k = 1$, the nearest data to the missing values are searched and the values of the nearest data are used to complement the missing values. If the nearest data also have missing values, the next nearest data without missing values are chosen instead.

2.4. Physical Activity Prediction Model Using an Autoencoder

In this section, we first summarize how we constructed a neural network for physical activity. There were two steps for the construction. The type of neural network trained in the first step was an "autoencoder". The autoencoder was constructed so as to extract important information from the inputs (test items). This was called "pre-training". Then, in the second step, a simple "feed-forward neural network" was constructed by changing the neural network structure built in step 1 to predict physical activity levels. This was called "fine-tuning".

Then, 3- and 4-layer neural networks (NNs) were used to build prediction models and each model was constructed using a combination of pre-training with the autoencoder and fine-tuning. The autoencoder was composed of an encoder, which converted the inputs into feature values, and a decoder, which reconstructed the inputs based on the obtained feature values. The goal of the pre-training was to set the initial weights of the NNs for the training that made the inputs and outputs coincide. The pre-training had the effect of constructing an effective encoder that extracted features that were hidden in the test items. Following pre-training, fine-tuning was conducted to achieve the final objective, i.e., the prediction of T-Ex.

Figure 1 shows the 3-layer autoencoder that conducted the pre-training. Figure 2 shows the model structure used for the fine-tuning, which was constructed after pre-training. In Figure 1, the number of input units was 34, where 32 units corresponded to the test items (except T-Ex) and two units corresponded to T-Ex1 and T-Ex2. The number of output units was also 34, corresponding to the number of input units. There were two T-Ex units to represent the one-hot vectors for normal and abnormal activity, i.e., the normal case was represented as (T-Ex1, T-Ex2) = (1,0), while the abnormal case was represented as (T-Ex1, T-Ex2) = (0,1). The loss function used in the autoencoder training was the mean squared error (MSE).

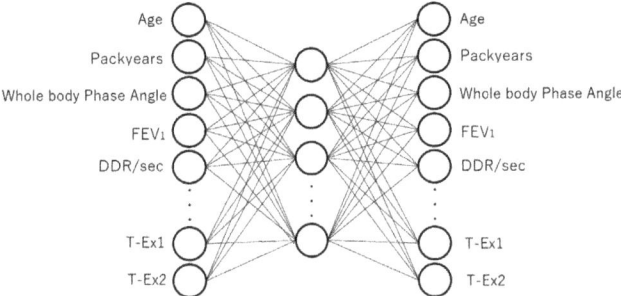

Figure 1. The model structure of the 3-layer autoencoder used for pre-training. There were 34 units in the input layer. In the hidden layer, a feature vector (feature values) that encoded the inputs was obtained. There were 34 units in the output layer, in which the inputs were reconstructed from the hidden layer vectors. The number of units in the hidden layer was 20, i.e., the feature values were represented by 20-dimensional vectors.

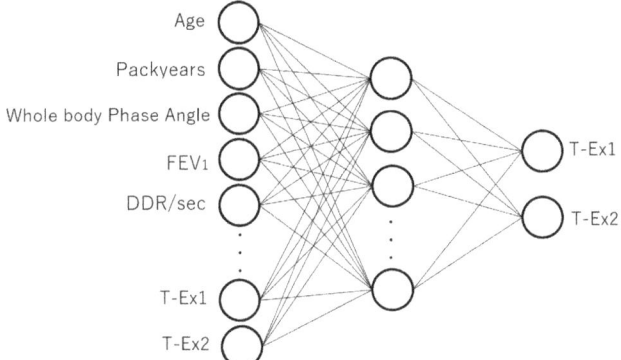

Figure 2. The model structure used for the fine-tuning, which was constructed after pre-training with the 3-layer autoencoder. The output layer in Figure 1 was removed and the model was connected to a new output layer to predict T-Ex1 and T-Ex2.

Next, a classifier was constructed using the autoencoder (Figure 2) to conduct fine-tuning. As the goal was to predict T-Ex, T-Ex could not be used as an input at this stage. Accordingly, when conducting fine-tuning, zeros were used as the inputs for the units corresponding to T-Ex. The two units in the output layer produced the respective probability that the input was normal or abnormal. The loss function used for fine-tuning was cross-entropy. Note that the weights of the input and hidden layers were adjusted in pre-training and further updated in fine-tuning.

For comparison, we also constructed a model based on a 4-layer autoencoder. The 4-layer autoencoder and the structure for fine-tuning are shown in Figures 3 and 4, respectively. The numbers of input and output units were the same as in the 3-layer case, while there were 20 units in both the first and second hidden layers. Representation ability increases with the number of neural network layers; however, because the amount of treated data was limited in this study, it was possible that overfitting could occur simply by deepening the number of layers. To prevent this overfitting, dropout [23] was applied to the first and second layers of the autoencoder (the dropout rate was 20% for the first layer and 10% for the second layer).

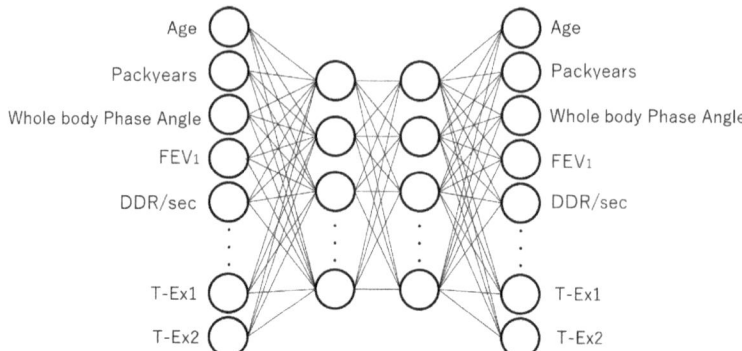

Figure 3. The model structure of the 4-layer autoencoder used for pre-training. The input layer had 34 units. In the two hidden layers, the vectors (feature values) that encoded the inputs were obtained. The output layer had 34 units and the inputs were reconstructed from the hidden layer vectors.

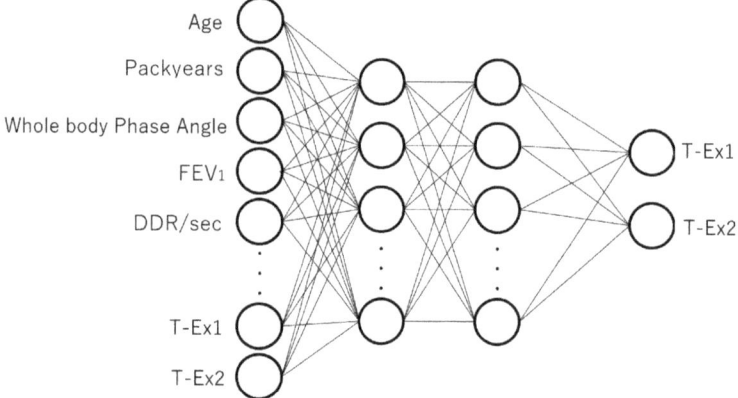

Figure 4. The model structure used for fine-tuning, which was constructed after pre-training with the 4-layer autoencoder. The output layer in Figure 3 was removed and the model was connected to a new output layer to predict T-Ex1 and T-Ex2.

2.5. Calculating the Importance of Each Test Item

Permutation importance [3] was used to calculate the importance of each test item. Permutation importance is a method of randomly substituting feature values between data. Using this process, the substituted feature values stop correlating with the response variable, that is, they lose their ability to explain the response variable. By comparing the accuracy when using the substituted data ($acc_{substitute}$) and the accuracy prior to substitution ($acc_{original}$), we could calculate to what extent the feature values contributed to the prediction. The importance of a test item was calculated using Equation (1).

$$importance(i) = acc_{original}(i) - acc_{substitute}(i), \tag{1}$$

where i is a test item with values that have been substituted to calculate its importance.

3. Evaluation Metrics and Results

3.1. Evaluation Metrics

In this section, we explain the method for separating the dataset into training and testing datasets. Here, the word "testing" is used to represent the testing dataset, while "test" is used for medical tests. The data used in this study included test results for the same patients on different days. Separating the dataset without taking this into account produced the possibility that test results from the same patient were included in both the training and testing datasets. As reliable prediction results could not be obtained in such cases, we ensured that data from the same patient were not included in either the training or testing datasets. Performance was then assessed using 20-fold cross-validation.

3.2. Prediction Accuracy of Each Method

Pairing datasets processed using one of the three missing value imputation methods with one of the four types of neural networks (NNs) (i.e., 3- and 4-layer NNs without pre-training and those with pre-training) yielded a total of 12 condition patterns. The mean accuracy for each method is shown in Table 2. The 3-layer NN that was pre-trained with missing values processed using MICE (3-layer NN with PT (MICE)) had the highest accuracy of 73.00%. In addition, focusing on missing value processing, MICE yielded the highest prediction accuracy compared to zero-padding ($p = 0.00025$) and kNN ($p = 0.023$). Conventionally, XGBoost [24] is often used in the analysis of table data; thus, a comparison between XGBoost, MICE, and the proposed method was also conducted. The accuracy of the proposed method was 73.00%, which was higher than that of XGBoost (66.12%) with a significant difference ($p = 0.016$). Therefore, the 3-layer NN with PT (MICE), i.e., the method with the highest accuracy, was used for the subsequent experiments.

Table 2. The mean accuracy obtained by each method. The 3-layer NN with PT (MICE) showed the highest accuracy.

Method	Accuracy (%)
3-layer NN without PT (zero-padding)	68.44
3-layer NN without PT (MICE)	72.55
3-layer NN without PT (kNN)	70.32
4-layer NN without PT (zero-padding)	65.98
4-layer NN without PT (MICE)	72.66
4-layer NN without PT (kNN)	69.74
3-layer NN with PT (zero-padding)	68.05
3-layer NN with PT (MICE)	73.00
3-layer NN with PT (kNN)	71.52
4-layer NN with PT (zero-padding)	67.63
4-layer NN with PT (MICE)	72.81
4-layer NN with PT (KNN)	70.05

Note: PT, pre-training.

3.3. Importance of Each Test Item

We calculated the permutation importance of each test item. In Figure 5, the importance of each test item is shown in a box plot. The triangles show the mean values and the test items are sorted by their mean values. Table 1 shows detailed information about the data statistics and their importance. In Table 1, the items are listed in order of importance. As previously stated, larger importance values indicated more important test items. In Figure 5, it can be seen that sex, the number of cigarettes per day, age, whole body phase angle, DDR, mMRC, FEV_1, %RV/TLC, pack years, and BNP were the most important test items (in this order). Interestingly, whole body phase angle (nutrition status) was the fourth most important test item. Test items showing an importance of 0 or less did not contribute to the prediction or could have been noise due to the effects of individual differences. The lifestyles of the patients also influenced their physical activity, so large deviations in importance were also found for some test items.

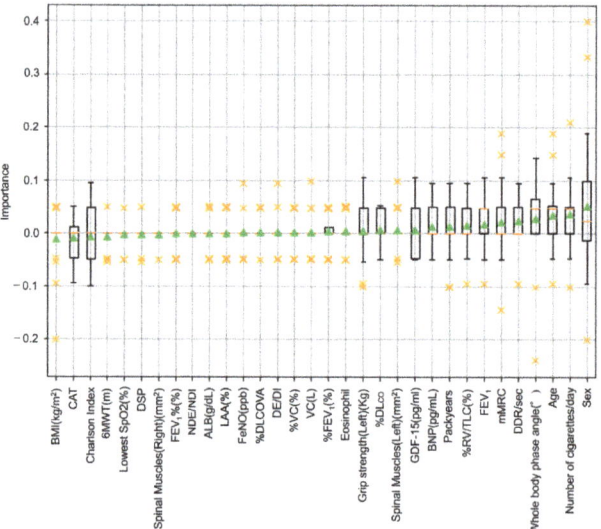

Figure 5. The importance of each test item. The horizontal axis shows the test items and the vertical axis shows their importance. The test items in order of effect on prediction performance were sex, the number of cigarettes per day, age, whole body phase angle, DDR, mMRC, FEV_1, %RV/TLC, pack years, and BNP.

3.4. Comparison of Classification Performance by the Number of Items Used

Making it possible to predict physical activity not only in large hospitals but also in regional clinics could contribute to the treatment of COPD by reducing test costs. Accordingly, to ascertain whether it would be possible to perform predictions using a smaller number of test items, we also inspected how classification performance changed as the number of test items decreased. Below are the five conditions that were used for this investigation.

1. 32 items (all of the test items);
2. 28 items (removing blood test);
3. 19 items (removing blood test and lung function test);
4. 15 items (removing blood test, lung function test, and walking test);
5. 10 items (removing blood test, lung function test, walking test, and chest imaging test).

Condition 1 was the case in which all 32 test items were used, while conditions 2 to 5 removed the blood test, lung function test, walking test, and chest imaging test one by one. Note that the items removed from conditions 2 to 5 were determined by referencing the items with the lowest importance in Figure 5 and considering the costs of the tests.

Table 3 shows the accuracy, precision, sensitivity, and specificity of each condition. As expected, the highest accuracy, precision, sensitivity, and specificity were obtained when all 32 items were used. However, even in condition 5, an accuracy of 69.28% was obtained, that is, the difference between conditions 1 and 5 was 3.72%. The test items used in condition 5 were age, sex, BMI, whole body phase angle, grip strength (left hand), Charlson index, pack years, the number of cigarettes per day, CAT, and mMRC. The p-values between the accuracy of condition 1 and the accuracy of the other conditions did not show any significant differences; therefore, a smaller number of test items could be conducted in ordinary clinical practice for the screening of physical activity disorder.

Table 3. The classification performance using different numbers of test items. The classifier using all 32 items showed the best accuracy, precision, sensitivity, and specificity. On the other hand, even when the number of test items was reduced to 10, the accuracy was still approximately 69%. The p-values show the results of t-tests on accuracy between condition 1 and the other conditions and demonstrate that there were no significant differences.

# of Items	Accuracy	Precision	Sensitivity	Specificity	p-Value (vs. Condition 1)
32	73.00	75.34	76.59	69.40	–
28	70.78	73.07	73.49	67.79	0.178
19	69.42	70.23	72.64	69.10	0.106
15	69.05	72.09	73.66	67.65	0.055
10	69.28	71.09	73.66	67.08	0.182

3.5. Sensitivity of T-Ex by Range

In this study, all T-Ex values of less than 3 were classified as abnormal, but a T-Ex value of less than 1.5 is defined as physical inactivity and implies a poor prognosis [25]. As a result, for patients with T-Ex values of 1.5 or less, there is a particularly prioritized need for physicians to respond, so it would be preferable to be able to predict these values without overlooking any cases. Accordingly, in this section, we analyze the sensitivity of T-Ex by range (Table 4). The analysis was performed using a prediction model for all 32 items. In this investigation, cases were divided into $2.5 \leq$ T-Ex < 3.0, $2.0 \leq$ T-Ex < 2.5, $1.5 \leq$ T-Ex < 2.0, and T-Ex < 1.5 and the sensitivity was calculated for each range. As can be seen from Table 4, the number of cases in which $2.5 \leq$ T-Ex < 3.0 was 217, of which 166 cases were correctly predicted to be abnormal with a sensitivity of 76.50%. The sensitivity for $2.0 \leq$ T-Ex < 2.5 was 79.46%, while that for $1.5 \leq$ T-Ex < 2.0 was 85.62% and that for T-Ex < 1.5 (severe physical activity reduction) was 89.36%. The sensitivity increased for patients with lower T-Ex values, indicating that the trained model captured the features of physically inactive patients.

Table 4. The sensitivity by T-Ex range. TP (true positive) represents the number of correctly predicted positive cases as positive and FN (false negative) represents the number of incorrectly predicted positive cases as negative. Therefore, TP + FN represents the actual positive numbers. Sensitivity was calculated using TP/(TP + FN).

	$2.5 \leq$ T-Ex < 3.0	$2.0 \leq$ T-Ex < 2.5	$1.5 \leq$ T-Ex < 2.0	T-Ex < 1.5
TP	166	147	125	84
TP + FN	217	185	146	94
Sensitivity (%)	76.50	79.46	85.62	89.36

3.6. Classification Performance for Healthy Individuals, Non-COPD Patients, and COPD Patients

We also analyzed the classification performance for healthy individuals, non-COPD patients, and COPD patients (Table 5). To obtain these results, the same trained model was used for all three patient categories. Note that the data to be predicted did not provide the model with any information regarding which category the patients belonged to.

Table 5. The classification performance for healthy individuals, non-COPD patients, and COPD patients.

	Accuracy (%)	Precision (%)	Sensitivity (%)	Specificity (%)
Healthy Individuals	88.00	0.00	0.00	100.0
Non-COPD Patients	68.49	70.27	65.00	72.03
COPD Patients	78.32	77.88	93.62	48.98

As shown in Table 5, extreme values for sensitivity (0%) and specificity (100%) were found for healthy individuals. Table 6 shows a confusion matrix of the classification results for healthy individuals, for which only three positive cases were found in the dataset. Accordingly, it is possible that training was insufficient due to the lack of positive cases among the healthy individuals. It is also possible that the test results obtained for healthy individuals rarely showed any signs of physical activity reduction.

The predictions for COPD and non-COPD patients, as shown in Table 5, had high sensitivity and low specificity, which was contrary to the results for healthy individuals. Therefore, the features of positive cases were captured well. In the test results for COPD patients and non-COPD patients, the characteristics of positive cases were strongly expressed, while it was more difficult to make negative classifications. Tables 7 and 8 show the confusion matrices of the classification results for COPD patients and non-COPD patients, respectively. For patients with COPD, out of the 94 actual positive cases, 89 cases were correctly classified as positive. For non-COPD patients, out of the 120 actual positive cases, 94 cases were correctly classified as positive, indicating a weaker expression of features for reduced physical activity in comparison to that for COPD patients.

Table 6. The confusion matrix of the classification results for healthy individuals.

		Prediction Positive	Negative
Actual	Positive	0	3
	Negative	0	22

Table 7. The confusion matrix of the classification results for COPD patients.

		Prediction Positive	Negative
Actual	Positive	88	6
	Negative	25	24

Table 8. The confusion matrix of the classification results for non-COPD patients.

		Prediction Positive	Negative
Actual	Positive	78	42
	Negative	33	85

4. Discussion

In this study, test results from patients with respiratory illnesses, including COPD, who were examined at the Yamaguchi University Hospital in Japan were used to construct a physical activity prediction model. An analysis was performed to determine which test items were important for predicting physical activity. While this study shared the same goal as previous studies in terms of the prediction of physical activity, we aimed to use a different motivation and technical approach. First, if physical activity could be predicted using simple tests that could be conducted in daily clinical practice, the efficiency of COPD treatment could be improved, even in areas with limited medical resources. Second, we implemented two measures to increase the applicability of machine learning to insufficient datasets. The first measure was the enhancement of the amount of data using missing value imputation. As it is difficult to conduct all possible tests on all patients, many missing values were included in the dataset. Accordingly, the following three missing value imputation methods were applied to enhance the data: zero-padding, MICE, and kNN. The second measure was the enhancement of feature extraction through the pre-training of the neural network using an autoencoder. By extracting useful information from test items measured during ordinary clinical practice, we strove to improve the performance of our prediction model for physical activity using machine learning. The results of our experiments indicated that the neural network that was pre-trained using the autoencoder with missing value imputation performed using MICE was the most effective model. Sex, the number of cigarettes per day, age, and whole body phase angle were the most important test items. This implied that it could be possible to conduct screening for reduced physical activity using some low-cost test items while omitting other tests, such as pulmonary function tests. Moreover, the fact that whole body phase angle was a useful item allowed us to infer that poor nutritional status could be related to poor prognosis accompanying physical inactivity. This suggests that in the future, there could be a need to longitudinally examine whether nutrition treatment interventions are effective as new methods of treatment for physical activity disorder. Although there have been studies attempting to find relationships between COPD patients and physical activity/muscle strength/body composition using whole body phase angle [26–28], to date, multifactorial analysis using machine learning, including blood, lung function, walking, and chest imaging tests, has not been performed. Therefore, this study showed that whole body phase angle was an important indicator for predicting physical activity.

This study had several limitations. First, there is room for improvement in the accuracy of 73.00%. As the amount of physical activity among patients is related to their personality and environment, it is difficult to obtain accurate predictions based solely on clinical test results. Further improvements in prediction performance may be aided by the collection of new data obtained via questionnaires concerning the living environments of patients. However, the prediction sensitivity for T-Ex < 1.5 was 89.36%, a level that could be clinically helpful as a screening method for reduction in physical activity. Furthermore, when calculating the importance of the test items, we only focused on single items to determine how much they contributed to the classification. If several highly correlated feature values existed, it could be possible that some truly important items were regarded as less important as the information could be imputed from other items, even with the removal of important items. Accordingly, it may be possible to extract the truly important items by calculating item importance after simultaneously shuffling highly correlated items. From another perspective, by changing combinations when shuffling multiple items, it may be possible to discover that although certain items have a small effect on classification, they could have a large effect when combined with other items. Additionally, only one type of data from Yamaguchi University Hospital was used in this study. However, the proposed model is universally applicable to table-form datasets, including those with missing values; thus, we will apply it to other datasets and evaluate its performance.

Author Contributions: All authors directly participated in the preparation of this manuscript. Y.N. and S.M. contributed to the construction of the models, the experiments, and the writing of the manuscript; T.H., Y.M., K.D., A.F.-C. and K.M. contributed to the data analysis, the discussion of the results, and the writing of the manuscript. All authors have read and agreed to the published version of the manuscript.

Funding: This work was supported by grants from JSPS KAKENHI (JP22K12152, JP21K07675, and JP19K12120). The funder had no role in the design, conduct, or reporting of this work.

Institutional Review Board Statement: This study was approved by the Institutional Review Board of Yamaguchi University Hospital (H27-204) and was conducted according to the principles of the Declaration of Helsinki.

Informed Consent Statement: Informed consent was obtained from all individuals included in this study.

Data Availability Statement: The dataset used in this study is not publicly available due to ethical constraints.

Acknowledgments: We would also like to thank Hiroe Hotta for helping with the data collection.

Conflicts of Interest: The authors declare no conflict of interest.

References

1. Cooper, C.B. Airflow obstruction and exercise. *Respir. Med.* **2009**, *103*, 325–334. [CrossRef] [PubMed]
2. Waschki, B.; Kirsten, A.; Holz, O.; Müller, K.C.; Meyer, T.; Watz, H.; Magnussen, H. Physical Activity Is the Strongest Predictor of All-Cause Mortality in Patients With COPD: A Prospective Cohort Study. *Chest* **2011**, *140*, 331–342. [CrossRef] [PubMed]
3. Troosters, T.; van der Molen, T.; Polkey, M.; Rabinovich, R.A.; Vogiatzis, I.; Weisman, I.; Kulich, K. Improving physical activity in COPD: Towards a new paradigm. *Respir. Res.* **2013**, *14*, 115. [CrossRef]
4. Hirano, T.; Doi, K.; Matsunaga, K.; Takahashi, S.; Donishi, T.; Suga, K.; Oishi, K.; Yasuda, K.; Mimura, Y.; Harada, M.; et al. A Novel Role of Growth Differentiation Factor (GDF)-15 in Overlap with Sedentary Lifestyle and Cognitive Risk in COPD. *J. Clin. Med.* **2020**, *9*, 2737. [CrossRef] [PubMed]
5. Matsunaga, K.; Harada, M.; Suizu, J.; Oishi, K.; Asami-Noyama, M.; Hirano, T. Comorbid Conditions in Chronic Obstructive Pulmonary Disease: Potential Therapeutic Targets for Unmet Needs. *J. Clin. Med.* **2020**, *9*, 3078. [CrossRef]
6. Ahmed, M.U.; Loutfi, A. Physical Activity Identification using Supervised Machine Learning and based on Pulse Rate. *Int. J. Adv. Comput. Sci. Appl.* **2013**, *4*, 209–217. [CrossRef]
7. Ahmadi, M.N.; Pavey, T.G.; Trost, S.G. Machine Learning Models for Classifying Physical Activity in Free-Living Preschool Children. *Sensors* **2020**, *20*, 4364. [CrossRef]
8. Mesanza, A.B.; Lucas, S.; Zubizarreta, A.; Cabanes, I.; Portillo, E.; Rodriguez-Larrad, A. A Machine Learning Approach to Perform Physical Activity Classification Using a Sensorized Crutch Tip. *IEEE Access* **2020**, *8*, 210023–210034. [CrossRef]
9. Alexos, A.; Moustakidis, S.; Kokkotis, C.; Tsaopoulos, D. Physical Activity as a Risk Factor in the Progression of Osteoarthritis: A Machine Learning Perspective. In *Proceedings of the Learning and Intelligent Optimization*; Kotsireas, I.S.; Pardalos, P.M., Eds.; Springer International Publishing: Cham, Swizerland, 2020; pp. 16–26.
10. Romain, A.J.; Horwath, C.; Bernard, P. Prediction of Physical Activity Level Using Processes of Change From the Transtheoretical Model: Experiential, Behavioral, or an Interaction Effect? *Am. J. Health Promot.* **2018**, *32*, 16–23. PMID: 29214837. [CrossRef]
11. Kim, J.C.; Chung, K. Prediction model of user physical activity using data characteristics-based long short-term memory recurrent neural networks. *KSII Trans. Internet Inf. Syst. (TIIS)* **2019**, *13*, 2060–2077.
12. Kawagoshi, A.; Iwakura, M.; Furukawa, Y.; Sugawara, K.; Takahashi, H.; Shioya, T. Prediction of Low-intensity Physical Activity in Stable Patients with Chronic Obstructive Pulmonary Disease. *Phys. Ther. Res.* **2022**, *25*, 143–149. [CrossRef]
13. Azuma, Y.; Minakata, Y.; Kato, M.; Tanaka, M.; Murakami, Y.; Sasaki, S.; Kawabe, K.; Ono, H. Validation of Simple Prediction Equations for Step Count in Japanese Patients with Chronic Obstructive Pulmonary Disease. *J. Clin. Med.* **2022**, *11*, 5535. [CrossRef]
14. Cleland, V.; Dwyer, T.; Venn, A. Which domains of childhood physical activity predict physical activity in adulthood? A 20-year prospective tracking study. *Br. J. Sport. Med.* **2012**, *46*, 595–602. Available online: https://bjsm.bmj.com/content/46/8/595.full.pdf (accessed on 1 March 2023). [CrossRef]
15. Glenmark, B.; Hedberg, G.; Jansson, E. Prediction of physical activity level in adulthood by physical characteristics, physical performance and physical activity in adolescence: an 11-year follow-up study. *Eur. J. Appl. Physiol. Occup. Physiol.* **1994**, *69*, 530–538. [CrossRef]
16. Rothney, M.P.; Schaefer, E.V.; Neumann, M.M.; Choi, L.; Chen, K.Y. Validity of Physical Activity Intensity Predictions by ActiGraph, Actical, and RT3 Accelerometers. *Obesity* **2008**, *16*, 1946–1952. Available online: https://onlinelibrary.wiley.com/doi/pdf/10.1038/oby.2008.279 (accessed on 1 March 2023). [CrossRef]
17. Zakariya, N.; Mohd Rosli, M. Physical activity prediction using fitness data: Challenges and issues. *Bull. Electr. Eng. Inform.* **2021**, *10*, 419–426. [CrossRef]
18. Murata, Y.; Hirano, T.; Doi, K.; Fukatsu-Chikumoto, A.; Hamada, K.; Oishi, K.; Kakugawa, T.; Yano, M.; Matsunaga, K. Computed Tomography Lung Density Analysis: An Imaging Biomarker Predicting Physical Inactivity in Chronic Obstructive Pulmonary Disease: A Pilot Study. *J. Clin. Med.* **2023**, *12*, 2959. [CrossRef]
19. Goodfellow, I.; Bengio, Y.; Courville, A. *Deep Learning*; MIT Press: Cambridge, MA, USA, 2016. Available online: http://www.deeplearningbook.org (accessed on 1 March 2023).
20. Hirano, T.; Matsunaga, K.; Hamada, K.; Uehara, S.; Suetake, R.; Yamaji, Y.; Oishi, K.; Asami, M.; Edakuni, N.; Ogawa, H.; et al. Combination of assist use of short-acting beta-2 agonists inhalation and guidance based on patient-specific restrictions in daily behavior: Impact on physical activity of Japanese patients with chronic obstructive pulmonary disease. *Respir. Investig.* **2019**, *57*, 133–139. [CrossRef]
21. Azur, M.J.; Stuart, E.A.; Frangakis, C.; Leaf, P.J. Multiple imputation by chained equations: What is it and how does it work? *Int. J. Methods Psychiatr. Res.* **2011**, *20*, 40–49. Available online: https://onlinelibrary.wiley.com/doi/pdf/10.1002/mpr.329 (accessed on 1 March 2023). [CrossRef]
22. Han, J.; Pei, J.; Tong, H. *Data Mining: Concepts and Techniques*; Morgan Kaufmann: Burlington, MA, USA, 2022.
23. Srivastava, N.; Hinton, G.; Krizhevsky, A.; Sutskever, I.; Salakhutdinov, R. Dropout: A Simple Way to Prevent Neural Networks from Overfitting. *J. Mach. Learn. Res.* **2014**, *15*, 1929–1958.
24. Chen, T.; Guestrin, C. XGBoost: A Scalable Tree Boosting System. In *Proceedings of the 22nd ACM SIGKDD International Conference on Knowledge Discovery and Data Mining*; Association for Computing Machinery: New York, NY, USA, 2016; KDD '16, p. 785–794. [CrossRef]

25. Haskell, W.L.; Lee, I.M.; Pate, R.R.; Powell, K.E.; Blair, S.N.; Franklin, B.A.; Macera, C.A.; Heath, G.W.; Thompson, P.D.; Bauman, A. Physical activity and public health: Updated recommendation for adults from the American College of Sports Medicine and the American Heart Association. *Circulation* **2007**, *116*, 1081. [CrossRef] [PubMed]
26. Zanella, P.B.; Àvila, C.C.; Chaves, F.C.; Gazzana, M.B.; Berton, D.C.; Knorst, M.M.; de Souza, C.G. Phase Angle Evaluation of Lung Disease Patients and Its Relationship with Nutritional and Functional Parameters. *J. Am. Coll. Nutr.* **2021**, *40*, 529–534. PMID: 32780649. [CrossRef] [PubMed]
27. Custódio Martins, P.; de Lima, T.R.; Silva, A.M.; Santos Silva, D.A. Association of phase angle with muscle strength and aerobic fitness in different populations: A systematic review. *Nutrition* **2022**, *93*, 111489. [CrossRef] [PubMed]
28. Martínez-Luna, N.; Orea-Tejeda, A.; González-Islas, D.; Flores-Cisneros, L.; Keirns-Davis, C.; Sánchez-Santillán, R.; Pérez-García, I.; Gastelum-Ayala, Y.; Martínez-Vázquez, V.; Martínez-Reyna, Ó. Association between body composition, sarcopenia and pulmonary function in chronic obstructive pulmonary disease. *BMC Pulm. Med.* **2022**, *22*, 106. [CrossRef]

Disclaimer/Publisher's Note: The statements, opinions and data contained in all publications are solely those of the individual author(s) and contributor(s) and not of MDPI and/or the editor(s). MDPI and/or the editor(s) disclaim responsibility for any injury to people or property resulting from any ideas, methods, instructions or products referred to in the content.

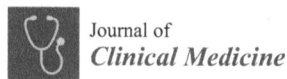

Article

Utility of the Shortness of Breath in Daily Activities Questionnaire (SOBDA-Q) to Detect Sedentary Behavior in Patients with Chronic Obstructive Pulmonary Disease (COPD)

Yoshikazu Yamaji [1], Tsunahiko Hirano [1], Hiromasa Ogawa [2], Ayumi Fukatsu-Chikumoto [1], Kazuki Matsuda [1], Kazuki Hamada [1], Shuichiro Ohata [1], Ryo Suetake [1], Yoriyuki Murata [1], Keiji Oishi [1], Maki Asami-Noyama [1], Nobutaka Edakuni [1], Tomoyuki Kakugawa [3] and Kazuto Matsunaga [1,*]

[1] Department of Respiratory Medicine and Infectious Disease, Graduate School of Medicine, Yamaguchi University, Ube 755-8505, Japan; yyamaji@yamaguchi-u.ac.jp (Y.Y.); tsuna@yamaguchi-u.ac.jp (T.H.); chiku05@yamaguchi-u.ac.jp (A.F.-C.); k0m1a2t8s1u1d2a1@gmail.com (K.M.); khamada@yamaguchi-u.ac.jp (K.H.); j015ebponyou@gmail.com (S.O.); rsuetake@yamaguchi-u.ac.jp (R.S.); yomurata@yamaguchi-u.ac.jp (Y.M.); ohishk@yamaguchi-u.ac.jp (K.O.); noyamama@yamaguchi-u.ac.jp (M.A.-N.); edakuni@yamaguchi-u.ac.jp (N.E.)

[2] Department of Occupational Health, Graduate School of Medicine, Tohoku University, Sendai 980-8575, Japan; ogawa-hiro@med.tohoku.ac.jp

[3] Department of Pulmonology and Gerontology, Graduate School of Medicine, Yamaguchi University, Ube 755-8505, Japan; tomoyukikakugawa@gmail.com

* Correspondence: kazmatsu@yamaguchi-u.ac.jp; Tel.: +81-836-85-3123

Abstract: Sedentary behavior has been shown to be an independent predictor of mortality in patients with chronic obstructive pulmonary disease (COPD). However, physicians have difficulty ascertaining patients' activity levels because they tend to avoid shortness of breath. The reformed shortness of breath (SOB) in the daily activities questionnaire (SOBDA-Q) specifies the degree of SOB by measuring low-intensity activity behavior in everyday living. Therefore, we aimed to explore the utility of the SOBDA-Q in detecting sedentary COPD. We compared the modified Medical Research Council dyspnea scale (mMRC), COPD assessment test (CAT), and SOBDA-Q with physical activity levels (PAL) in 17 healthy patients, 32 non-sedentary COPD patients (PAL ≥ 1.5 METs·h), and 15 sedentary COPD patients (PAL < 1.5 METs·h) in this cross-sectional study. CAT and all domains of the SOBDA-Q in all patients are significantly correlated with PAL, even after adjusting for age. The dietary domain has the highest specificity, and the outdoor activity domain has the highest sensitivity for detecting sedentary COPD. Combining these domains helped determine patients with sedentary COPD (AUC = 0.829, sensitivity = 1.00, specificity = 0.55). The SOBDA-Q is associated with PAL and could be a useful tool for determining patients with sedentary COPD. Moreover, eating and outing inactivity claims reflect sedentary behavior in patients with COPD.

Keywords: sedentary behavior; physical activity; patient-reported outcome measures (PROMs); chronic obstructive pulmonary disease (COPD)

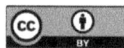

1. Introduction

Shortness of breath (SOB) on exertion is one of the most important symptoms and is said to accompany exercise intolerance and reduce physical activity in patients with chronic obstructive pulmonary disease (COPD) [1,2]. Patients with symptomatic COPD spend less time walking and standing and, consequently, tend to be sedentary compared to healthy patients [3]. Recent studies show that sedentary behavior is an independent predictor of mortality in patients with COPD [4,5]. However, it is difficult for physicians to identify sedentary behavior in patients using a standard questionnaire because patients with a sedentary lifestyle are more likely to avoid the discomfort of feeling SOB on exertion and tend to underreport their symptoms. Therefore, in a clinical setting, we subjectively assessed sedentary behavior as physical activity (PA) using questionnaires and objectively assessed PA using pedometers and accelerometers [6]. Although conventional PA-related questionnaires are inexpensive and easy to apply to patients, they are reported to be less sensitive than accelerometers, especially when assessing low-intensity physical activity, including sedentary behavior [6]. This could arise from inaccurate perception, recall of information by the subject, questionnaire design, age, and the cognitive ability of the patient [6]. The University of California, San Diego Shortness of Breath questionnaire (UCSD SOBQ) [7] is a specific daily life activity questionnaire that uses the verbal rating scale. We devised the SOB in the daily activities questionnaire (SOBDA-Q), which can detect detailed situations in which patients with COPD experience SOB in their daily lives. Therefore, we hypothesized that the SOBDA-Q could be a useful tool for detecting sedentary behavior in patients with COPD.

2. Materials and Methods

2.1. Study Subjects

This is a cross-sectional study. We recruited 17 healthy patients and 47 patients with COPD who were treated at Yamaguchi University Hospital between January 2017 and November 2020. Healthy patients were defined as those with no respiratory, cardiovascular, or musculoskeletal diseases that interfered with their daily lives. COPD was diagnosed by a respiratory physician in accordance with the Global Initiative for Chronic Obstructive Lung Disease (GOLD) guidelines and treated according to the GOLD guidelines [1]. Patients with COPD were stable and had no exacerbations for at least three months before the study. Patients with other pulmonary diseases, such as interstitial lung disease and bronchiectasis, or those with restricted physical activity due to complications, such as cardiac or neuromuscular disease, were excluded. The study protocol was explained to healthy patients and COPD patients, and written informed consent was obtained from all patients. This study was approved by the local ethics committee of Yamaguchi Medical University (IRB number:H27-204).

2.2. Evaluation of Physical Activity

An Active Style Pro HJA-750C® (Omron Healthcare Co., Ltd., Kyoto, Japan) with a triaxial acceleration sensor was attached to the waist, and physical activity was recorded continuously for 2 weeks. We measured the metabolic equivalent (METs) values and calculated the physical activity level (PAL) by multiplying the activity METs by the duration of the activity in hours (MET·h/day), as previously reported [8,9]. To obtain typical physical activity data, we collected values from weekdays without rain during the two weeks. The first and last days of recording were excluded because the data for one day were unavailable. Based on the 2011 Compendium of Physical Activity [10], we defined PAL < 1.5 METs as sedentary behavior [11], 1.6–2.9 METs as light-intensity activities [12], 3–5.9 METs as moderate-intensity activities, and ≥6 METs as vigorous-intensity activities. METs for various daily activities included approximately 1.3 METs for sitting and quietly watching TV, 2.0 METs for cooking and washing, 3.0 METs for walking the dog, 4.0 METs for climbing stairs, and 6.0 METs for bicycling. In addition, the American College of Sports Medicine and the American Heart Association recommend that older adults perform moderate-intensity (3 METs to 6 METs) aerobic exercise for at least 0.5 h five days a week [13]. Therefore, we considered patients with PAL < 1.5 METs·h as those with sedentary behavior [14]. In this study, we analyzed COPD groups with a PAL cutoff of <1.5 METs·h.

2.3. Assessment of Questionnaire Patient-Reported Outcome Measures (PROMs)

We used the modified Medical Research Council (mMRC) dyspnea scale, COPD assessment test (CAT), and SOBDA-Q as PROMs. The SOBDA-Q is a composite SOB questionnaire comprising 22 items organized into six domains of daily living (morning, dietary, indoor activity, outdoor activity, recreation, and night-time activity) (Table S1). The SOBDA-Q score was set using a scale with a minimum of one point (I do not do it because

I feel short of breath) and a maximum of six points (I'm doing as usual without adjusting. I don't feel short of breath). Activity items that were not originally performed were defined as "no evaluation." We calculated the average score for every domain except for the absence of evaluation. For example, if you scored 4 points for brushing teeth, 5 points for changing clothes, and 4 points for defecation/urination in the morning domain, the score for the morning domain would be calculated as (4 + 5 + 4)/3 items = 4.33 points (Table S2). This SOBDA-Q was devised and prepared by Dr. Hiromasa Ogawa, Tohoku University Hospital, with permission from the authors of the University of California, San Diego Shortness of Breath questionnaire (UCSD SOBQ) [7]. Trained research assistants administered the Japanese versions of the mMRC, CAT, and SOBDA-Q to participants.

2.4. Assessment of Pulmonary Function

Pulmonary function was assessed using a dry-rolling seal spirometer (CHESTAC-8800; Chest Co., Tokyo, Japan) according to the American Thoracic Society/European Respiratory Society recommendations [15].

2.5. Statistical Analysis

Data are shown as mean ± standard deviation. The chi-square test or Fisher's exact test was used to compare the categorical data. Wilcoxon's rank sum test was used to compare nonparametric data between each group. Spearman's rank correlation and multiple linear regression analyses using the least-squares method were performed to analyze the correlation between PAL and PROMs. We analyzed sensitivity versus specificity using the area under the curve (AUC) and found a cutoff value for PROMs that could detect COPD patients with PAL of <1.5 METs·h. Statistical analyses were performed using JMP Pro®, version 15.0.0 (SAS Institute, Inc., Cary, NC, USA). Statistical significance was set at $p < 0.05$.

3. Results

3.1. Patient Characteristics

The baseline patient characteristics are shown in Table 1. This study included 17 healthy patients, 32 non-sedentary patients with COPD, and 15 sedentary patients with COPD. A total of 43 patients with COPD (91.5%) were classified as GOLD stages 1 and 2; 17 patients with COPD (36.2%) had a CAT score <10 points; and 35 patients with COPD (74.5%) had mMRC grades 0 and 1. Compared to healthy patients, patients with COPD were significantly more likely to be male, older, and to have a higher smoking status, CAT score, mMRC grade, and severe airflow limitation ($p < 0.0001$, $p < 0.05$, $p < 0.0001$, $p < 0.0001$, $p < 0.05$, and $p < 0.05$, respectively).

3.2. Comparison of the Physical Activity among Patients

A comparison of PAL, duration of physical activity, and total number of steps among the patients is shown in Table 2. PAL, duration of physical activity at all activity intensities, and the total number of steps are significantly lower in sedentary patients with COPD across all groups. In particular, the duration of ≥2 METs in sedentary patients with COPD is significantly reduced to about half of that in non-sedentary patients with COPD (≥2 METs: 208.5 min vs. 93.8 min, $p < 0.0001$), and the duration of ≥3 METs and ≥4 METs in sedentary patients with COPD are significantly reduced to about one-quarter of that in non-sedentary patients with COPD (≥3 METs: 55.2 min vs. 14.7 min, $p < 0.0001$; ≥4 METs: 12.2 min vs. 2.7 min, $p < 0.0001$, respectively).

Table 1. Patient characteristics.

	HP (N = 17)	Non-Sedentary COPD (N = 32)	Sedentary COPD (N = 15)	p Value
Number, n (M/F)	4/13	32/0	14/1	<0.0001
Age (years)	61.1 ± 10.6	70.0 ± 8.0	70.9 ± 10.2	<0.05
BMI (kg/m^2)	21.8 ± 3.5	22.6 ± 2.8	24.9 ± 4.1	n.s.
Smoking status (non/ex/cu)	15/2/0	0/24/8	0/9/6	<0.0001
Smoking history (pack years)	3.6 ± 11.0	45.2 ± 26.7	51.8 ± 22.0	<0.0001
GOLD (1/2/3/4)	-	16/13/3/0	5/9/1/0	-
CAT (<10/≥10)	17/0	12/20	5/10	<0.0001
mMRC(0/1/2/3/4)	13/4/0/0/0	16/9/2/5/0	5/5/4/0/1	<0.05
FEV$_1$	2.38 ± 0.42	2.21 ± 0.56	1.90 ± 0.51	<0.05
%FEV$_1$	106.8 ± 12.6	77.7 ± 18.7	70.4 ± 16.0	<0.0001

Data are shown as means ± standard deviation. Abbreviations: HP, healthy patients; COPD, chronic obstructive pulmonary disease; BMI, body mass index; non, non-smoker; ex, ex-smoker; cu, current smoker; GOLD, Global Initiative for Chronic Obstructive Lung Disease; CAT, COPD assessment test; mMRC, modified Medical Research Council; FEV$_1$, forced expiratory volume in one second. p-value compared across all groups with the chi-square test or Fisher's exact test or the Wilcoxon test.

Table 2. Comparison of the physical activity among patients.

	HP (N = 17)	Non-Sedentary COPD (N = 32)	Sedentary COPD (N = 15)	p Value
PAL (METs·h)	5.18 ± 1.95 [a]	3.50 ± 1.99 [a]	0.87 ± 0.33	<0.0001
≥1METs (min)	776.1 ± 151.4 [b]	609.4 ± 180.9 [c]	495.5 ± 222.3	<0.0005
≥2METs (min)	259.8 ± 79.8 [a]	208.5 ± 87.2 [a]	93.8 ± 50.8	<0.0001
≥3METs (min)	83.9 ± 33.4 [a]	55.2 ± 31.3 [a]	14.7 ± 5.6	<0.0001
≥4METs (min)	20.2 ± 10.9 [a]	12.2 ± 14.6 [a]	2.7 ± 2.0	<0.0001
Total number of steps	6315.5 ± 2284.8 [a]	5224.7 ± 2860.0 [a]	1714.6 ± 1755.8	<0.0001

Data are shown as means ± standard deviation. Abbreviations: HP, healthy patients; COPD, chronic obstructive pulmonary disease; PAL, physical activity level; METs: metabolic equivalents; p-value compared across all groups with Wilcoxon test. [a] $p < 0.001$, [b] $p < 0.01$, [c] $p < 0.05$, in reference to sedentary COPD.

3.3. Comparison of PROMs among Patients

Table 3 shows a comparison of the mean scores for each PROMs among the patients. Significantly higher mMRC and CAT scores and lower SOBDA-Q scores in all domains are observed in sedentary patients with COPD. In particular, the average scores in the morning, dietary, outdoor activity, recreation, and night-time activity domains are significantly lower in sedentary patients with COPD to non-sedentary patients with COPD.

Table 3. Comparison of PROMs among patients.

	HP (N = 17)	Non-Sedentary COPD (N = 32)	Sedentary COPD (N = 15)	p Value
mMRC	0.2 ± 0.4 [b]	0.9 ± 1.1	1.1 ± 1.1	<0.05
CAT	4.1 ± 3.2 [a]	11.7 ± 6.7	15.4 ± 9.1	<0.0001
SOBDA-Q				
Morning	5.9 ± 0.2 [a]	5.5 ± 0.7 [c]	4.4 ± 1.5	<0.001
Dietary	5.9 ± 0.2 [a]	5.6 ± 0.8 [b]	4.3 ± 1.6	<0.0005
Indoor activity	5.9 ± 0.3 [b]	5.2 ± 1.0	4.3 ± 1.8	<0.05
Outdoor activity	6.0 ± 0.1 [a]	5.1 ± 1.1 [c]	3.8 ± 1.7	<0.0001
Recreation	5.6 ± 0.4 [a]	4.8 ± 1.1 [c]	3.7 ± 1.7	<0.0005
Night-time activity	5.9 ± 0.3 [c]	5.4 ± 0.9 [c]	4.3 ± 1.5	<0.001

Data are shown as means ± standard deviation. Abbreviations: HP, healthy patients; COPD, chronic obstructive pulmonary disease; mMRC, modified Medical Research Council; CAT, COPD assessment test; SOBDA-Q, shortness of breath in daily activities questionnaire. p-value compared across all groups with Wilcoxon test. [a] $p < 0.001$, [b] $p < 0.01$, [c] $p < 0.05$, in reference to sedentary COPD.

3.4. Correlation between PROMs and Physical Activity

The correlations between PROMs and PAL are presented in Table 4. MMRC and CAT show a significant moderate negative correlation with PAL in univariate analysis. All SOBDA-Q domains show significant positive correlations with PAL in the univariate analysis. The linear regression model adjusted for age using the least-squares method shows that the CAT and all SOBDA-Q domains have significant independent associations with PAL.

Table 4. Correlation between PROMs and physical activity in all patients.

Variables	Univariate Analysis		Multivariate Analysis	
	Correlation Coefficient (ρ)	p Value	Correlation Coefficient (F)	p Value
mMRC	−0.27	<0.05	0.25	n.s.
CAT	−0.42	<0.001	4.72	<0.05
SOBDA-Q				
Morning	0.48	<0.0001	5.46	<0.05
Dietary	0.6	<0.0001	5.5	<0.05
Indoor activity	0.44	<0.001	5.33	<0.05
Outdoor activity	0.62	<0.0001	6.28	<0.05
Recreation	0.44	<0.0005	4.23	<0.05
Night-time activity	0.44	<0.0005	5.04	<0.05

Univariate analysis was performed by Spearman's rank correlation coefficient. For multivariate analysis, multiple linear regression analysis using the least-squares method were performed to adjust correlation of univariate analysis by age. Abbreviations: n.s., not statistically significant.

3.5. The Relationship between Quartiles of PAL and PROMs

The relationship between quartiles of PAL (Q1: <1.6 METs·h, Q2: 1.6–3.0 METs·h, Q3: 3.0–4.5 METs·h, Q4: >4.5 METs·h) and mMRC, CAT, dietary, and outdoor activity domains of SOBDA-Q are shown in Figure 1. Significant differences are observed between the median values of Q1 and Q3 for CAT (13 vs. 5, $p < 0.05$). Similarly, the dietary domain shows significant differences between the median values of Q1, Q3, and Q4 (5 vs. 6, $p = 0.0005$, 5 vs. 6, $p < 0.005$, respectively) as well as between the median values of Q2 and Q3 or Q4 (5.75 vs. 6, $p < 0.01$, 5.75 vs. 6, $p < 0.05$, respectively). The outdoor activity domain shows significant differences between the median values of Q1, Q3, and Q4 (4.5 vs. 6, $p < 0.005$, 4.5 vs. 6, $p < 0.0005$, respectively).

3.6. The Diagnostic Ability of PROMs to Predict Sedentary Patients with COPD

We assessed the diagnostic ability of PROMs to predict sedentary patients with COPD using receiver operating characteristics (ROC) analysis (Table 5). The outdoor activity domain (cut off points ≤ 5.667) shows the highest area under the curve (AUC), and the dietary domain (cut off points ≤ 5.5) shows the second highest. Figure 2 shows the ROC curves for CAT (cut off points ≥ 21) and the SOBDA-Q combination for the two domains (outdoor activity and dietary). The ROC analysis of the SOBDA-Q combination for predicting COPD in sedentary patients has an AUC of 0.829, a sensitivity of 1.00, and a specificity of 0.55.

3.7. The Relationship between Stratified CAT, SOBDA-Q Combination, and PAL

Using the cutoff values obtained from ROC analysis, a scatter plot of the relationship between CAT, SOBDA-Q combination, and PAL is shown in Figure 3. Compared to the CAT score <21 group, the CAT score $\geq$21 group shows significantly less physical activity ($p < 0.005$). Compared with both negative groups of the SOBDA-Q combination (two domains negative), at least one domain-positive group (one domain positive or two domains positive) shows significantly less physical activity ($p < 0.05$, $p < 0.0001$, respectively). In particular, there are no sedentary patients with COPD who test negative in the two domains of the SOBDA-Q combination.

Table 5. Diagnostic ability in PROMs to predict sedentary patients with COPD.

Variables	AUC	Cut Off	Sensitivity	Specificity
mMRC	0.641	1	0.67	0.59
CAT	0.686	21	0.4	0.92
SOBDA-Q				
Morning	0.733	5	0.67	0.76
Dietary	0.759	5.5	0.67	0.8
Indoor activity	0.679	5	0.54	0.76
Outdoor activity	0.817	5.667	1	0.58
Recreation	0.755	4.667	0.67	0.76
Night-time activity	0.756	5.667	0.73	0.73

Abbreviations: mMRC, modified Medical Research Council; CAT, COPD assessment test; SOBDA, shortness of breath in daily activities questionnaire; AUC, area under the curve.

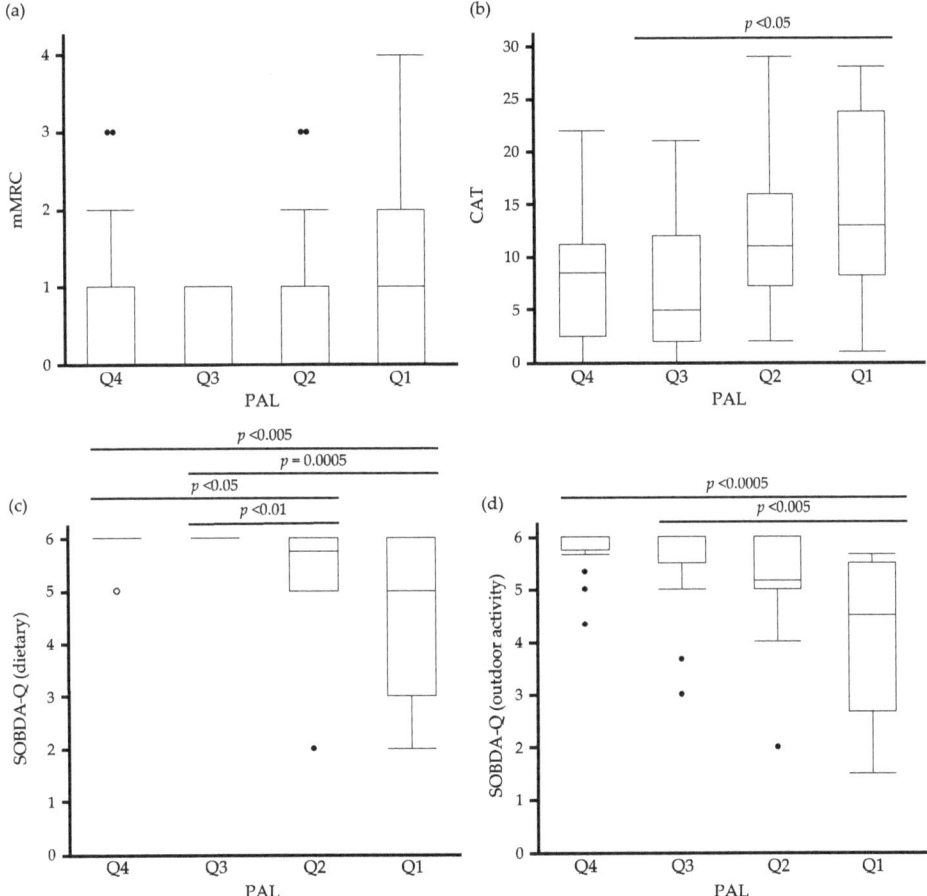

Figure 1. The relationship between quartiles of PAL and PROMs. (a) Box and whisker plots of PAL (quartiles) versus (a) mMRC, (b) CAT, (c) SOBDA-Q (dietary), and (d) SOBDA-Q (outdoor activity), where mMRC, CAT, and SOBDA-Q are represented by PAL (quartiles). Data are presented as the median and interquartile range (box), with minimum and maximum values (whiskers). Data beyond the end of the whiskers are called "outlying" points and are plotted individually. PROMs, patient-reported outcome measures; open circles, healthy patients; closed circles, COPD patients. Data were analyzed using the Wilcoxon test.

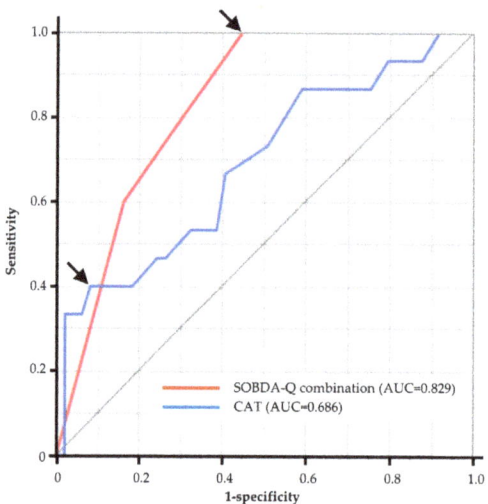

Figure 2. Diagnostic ability of CAT and SOBDA-Q combination to predict sedentary COPD. CAT, COPD assessment test; SOBDA-Q, Shortness of Breath in Daily Activities questionnaire; AUC, area under the curve. The arrow indicates the cut-off point.

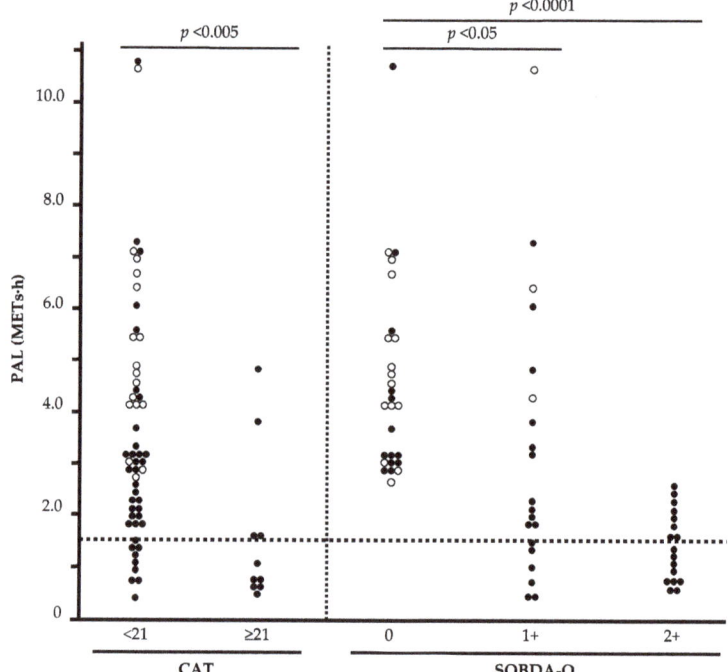

Figure 3. The relationship between stratified CAT, SOBDA-Q combination, and physical activity. CAT, COPD assessment test; SOBDA-Q, Shortness of Breath in Daily Activities questionnaire; open circles: healthy patients; closed circles: COPD patients. The dotted line represents 1.5 METs·h. Data were analyzed with the Wilcoxon test.

4. Discussion

We demonstrate that the newly devised SOBDA-Q significantly correlates with physical activity levels. Moreover, the combination of dietary- and outdoor-activity-related SOB can accurately identify patients with sedentary COPD.

The International Physical Activity questionnaire (IPAQ) [16] and its modified version, the Global Physical Activity questionnaire (GPAQ) [17], are representative physical activity questionnaires. They are not applied to patients with COPD but to the general adult population. They do not have sufficient sensitivity to detect low-intensity physical activity reduction [18], which is a feature of patients with COPD [3]. Meanwhile, the Minnesota Leisure Time Physical Activity questionnaire (Minnesota LTPA Questionnaire), the Baecke Questionnaire of Habitual Physical Activity, and the Physical Activity Scale in the Elderly (PASE) questionnaire are more valid in the older and other populations [6,19–21]. However, since many patients with COPD limit their daily activities to avoid experiencing dyspnea and underestimate the feeling of dyspnea by patients themselves [22], it is difficult for physicians to accurately analogize physical activity, especially daily physical activity, using the above self-reported questionnaires. We show that in the conventional subjective SOB evaluation questionnaire, the mMRC is poorly correlated with the objectively measured PAL and that the mMRC does not increase in a PAL-dependent manner (Table 4 and Figure 1). In short, the simple SOB questionnaire has limitations in assessing the physical activity of patients with COPD who tend to avoid daily activities [23–25].

CAT also did not have sufficient power to capture physical activity as sensitively as SOBDA-Q in this study. CAT includes major symptoms in patients with COPD [26]; however, some questions, such as cough, sputum, and sleep status, are not associated with physical activity. Furthermore, CAT is formatted as a semantic differential six-point scale [26], and it may require higher cognitive demands from participants owing to the abstract level of interpretation between the end-label representations [27]. In other words, the interpretation of each person's end-label scores differs depending on how each person sets the maximum end-label value. On the other hand, SOBDA-Q can reflect wide-intensity activities in various life situations and specifically determine the latent behavior that saves daily activities due to SOB. Therefore, as shown in Table 3, SOBDA-Q shows significant differences in mean scores not only between HP and sedentary patients with COPD, but also between non-sedentary patients and sedentary patients with COPD. We consider this detection ability to be a strength of SOBDA-Q. Additionally, SOBDA-Q indicates the degree of breathlessness in specific terms, making it easier for participants to choose their options without hesitation. Hence, as shown in Table 4 and Figure 1, SOBDA-Q may have resulted in more PAL-dependent changes than CAT.

Furthermore, within each SOBDA-Q domain, the dietary and outdoor activity domains are more important for detecting sedentary COPD (Tables 4 and 5). Meal-induced dyspnea in patients with COPD is thought to be related to irregular breathing caused due to chewing and swallowing [28,29], abdominal distension after eating [30], and upper extremity exertion during eating [31,32]. In addition, the causes of an outdoor-activity-related SOB in patients with COPD are thought to be related to increased respiratory rate and inspiratory time/total time ratio (Tin/Ttot) and end-expiratory load during a conversation [33–35]. However, the causal relationship is unclear, and further analysis is required to understand this mechanism.

The specific SOBDA-Q combination had high sensitivity (1.00) for detecting sedentary COPD (Figure 2). This means that asking patients with COPD questions related to dietary and outdoor activities would be useful as a screening tool for sedentary behavior. Although approximately 90% of the patients with COPD in this study had GOLD stages 1 and 2, approximately 30% had already been sedentary. This is consistent with previous studies in which COPD patients with GOLD stages 1 or 2 had reduced physical activity [3]. These results suggest that our SOBDA-Q is useful for detecting sedentary behavior in early-stage COPD and for initiating early intervention for COPD.

Regarding the clinical application of SOBDA-Q, Hirano et al. demonstrated that using SOBDA-Q as a guide for the assistive use of short-acting β2 agonists (SABA) can increase PAL in patients with COPD [36]. Using the SOBDA-Q as a communication tool in daily medical practice, medical staff (doctors, nurses, etc.) can recognize and understand patient-specific breathlessness situations and circumstances. Medical staff will be able to instruct patients with COPD in situations where they need assistive use of SABA. Patients with COPD can also access this tool to understand when and how to use assistive use of SABA. In particular, the SOBDA-Q can identify unrecognized inactivity, which has been restricted owing to potential SOB in daily life. This concept coincides with previous studies showing that behavioral change counseling is needed to improve physical inactivity [37]. We believe that the SOBDA-Q can be an interactive communication tool between medical staff and patients with COPD that promotes behavioral change.

However, there are several limitations in generalizing the results of this study. First, the sample size was small, and there was a difference in the ratio of male to female participants between healthy patients and patients with COPD. Some studies have reported sex differences in breathlessness and other symptoms in patients with COPD [38,39], which may have affected the results of this study. In addition, multivariate analysis including sex, smoking status, and pulmonary function as confounding factors could not be performed in this study because of lack of statistical power due to the small sample size. In the future, we will examine this issue with a large sample size. Second, many patients had early GOLD stage. As there may be differences in symptoms and physical activity according to the severity of airflow obstruction [40], further studies are needed to verify this by recruiting more patients with more severe stages. Third, the results were evaluated using the average score for each SOBDA-Q domain. Using the average score, we were able to compare the SOB in each daily lifestyle; however, some patients did not perform all daily physical activities in the domains. Fourth, we did not compare SOBDA-Q to questionnaires other than the mMRC or CAT. Therefore, we cannot mention any differences from other questionnaires. We will consider further studies that incorporate other questionnaires in the future. Fifth, we did not perform a combination analysis of the SOBDA-Q as a questionnaire for identifying sedentary patients with COPD. Therefore, the present study did not examine the effect of SOBDA-Q in combination with CAT or mMRC. Further studies will be conducted to increase the sample size and examine the usefulness of combining the SOBDA-Q with other questionnaires.

5. Conclusions

The newly developed SOBDA-Q correlates significantly with objectively measured physical activity and has the potential to accurately identify patients with sedentary COPD.

Supplementary Materials: The following supporting information can be downloaded at: https://www.mdpi.com/article/10.3390/jcm12124105/s1, Table S1: The Shortness of Breath in the Daily Activities questionnaire (SOBDA-Q); Table S2: The SOBDA-Q scoring method (example).

Author Contributions: Conceptualization, Y.Y., T.H., H.O. and K.M. (Kazuto Matsunaga); methodology, Y.Y., T.H., H.O. and K.M. (Kazuto Matsunaga); formal analysis, Y.Y. and T.H.; investigation, Y.Y. and T.H.; resources, Y.Y., T.H., H.O., A.F.-C., K.M. (Kazuki Matsuda), K.H., S.O., R.S., Y.M., K.O., M.A.-N., N.E., T.K. and K.M. (Kazuto Matsunaga); data curation, Y.Y. and T.H.; writing—original draft preparation, Y.Y., T.H. and K.M. (Kazuto Matsunaga); writing—review and editing, Y.Y., T.H., H.O., A.F.-C., K.M. (Kazuki Matsuda), K.H., S.O., R.S., Y.M., K.O., M.A.-N., N.E., T.K. and K.M. (Kazuto Matsunaga); project administration, Y.Y., T.H., H.O. and K.M. (Kazuto Matsunaga). All authors have read and agreed to the published version of the manuscript.

Funding: This research was was supported by a grant from the Japan Society for the Promotion of Science (JSPS) KAKENHI (grant number JP21K08180). The funder had no role in the design, conduct, or reporting of this work.

Institutional Review Board Statement: The study was conducted in accordance with the Declaration of Helsinki, and approved by the Institutional Review Board of Yamaguchi University Hospital (IRB number: H27-204).

Informed Consent Statement: Informed consent was obtained from all patients involved in the study.

Data Availability Statement: The data analyzed during the current study are included in this article. Additional data are available from the corresponding author upon request.

Acknowledgments: We thank Hiroe Hotta and Kumiko Teramoto and Keiko Doi for collecting patient data.

Conflicts of Interest: The authors declare no conflict of interest.

References

1. Global Initiative for Chronic Obstructive Lung Disease (GOLD). Global Strategy for the Diagnosis, Management, and Prevention of Chronic Obstructive Pulmonary Disease (2023 report). Available online: http://www.goldcopd.org/ (accessed on 10 February 2023).
2. Giacomini, M.; DeJean, D.; Simeonov, D.; Smith, A. Experiences of living and dying with COPD: A systematic review and synthesis of the qualitative empirical literature. *Ont. Health Technol. Assess. Ser.* **2012**, *12*, 1–47.
3. Pitta, F.; Troosters, T.; Spruit, M.A.; Probst, V.S.; Decramer, M.; Gosselink, R. Characteristics of physical activities in daily life in chronic obstructive pulmonary disease. *Am. J. Respir. Crit. Care Med.* **2005**, *171*, 972–977. [CrossRef] [PubMed]
4. Furlanetto, K.C.; Donaria, L.; Schneider, L.P.; Lopes, J.R.; Ribeiro, M.; Fernandes, K.B.; Hernandes, N.A.; Pitta, F. Sedentary Behavior Is an Independent Predictor of Mortality in Subjects With COPD. *Respir. Care* **2017**, *62*, 579–587. [CrossRef]
5. Waschki, B.; Kirsten, A.; Holz, O.; Muller, K.C.; Meyer, T.; Watz, H.; Magnussen, H. Physical activity is the strongest predictor of all-cause mortality in patients with COPD: A prospective cohort study. *Chest* **2011**, *140*, 331–342. [CrossRef]
6. Pitta, F.; Troosters, T.; Probst, V.S.; Spruit, M.A.; Decramer, M.; Gosselink, R. Quantifying physical activity in daily life with questionnaires and motion sensors in COPD. *Eur. Respir. J.* **2006**, *27*, 1040–1055. [CrossRef] [PubMed]
7. Eakin, E.G.; Resnikoff, P.M.; Prewitt, L.M.; Ries, A.L.; Kaplan, R.M. Validation of a new dyspnea measure: The UCSD Shortness of Breath Questionnaire. University of California, San Diego. *Chest* **1998**, *113*, 619–624. [CrossRef] [PubMed]
8. Sugino, A.; Minakata, Y.; Kanda, M.; Akamatsu, K.; Koarai, A.; Hirano, T.; Sugiura, H.; Matsunaga, K.; Ichinose, M. Validation of a compact motion sensor for the measurement of physical activity in patients with chronic obstructive pulmonary disease. *Respiration* **2012**, *83*, 300–307. [CrossRef]
9. Matthews, C.E.; Ainsworth, B.E.; Thompson, R.W.; Bassett, D.R., Jr. Sources of variance in daily physical activity levels as measured by an accelerometer. *Med. Sci. Sports Exerc.* **2002**, *34*, 1376–1381. [CrossRef]
10. Ainsworth, B.E.; Haskell, W.L.; Herrmann, S.D.; Meckes, N.; Bassett, D.R., Jr.; Tudor-Locke, C.; Greer, J.L.; Vezina, J.; Whitt-Glover, M.C.; Leon, A.S. 2011 Compendium of Physical Activities: A second update of codes and MET values. *Med. Sci. Sports Exerc.* **2011**, *43*, 1575–1581. [CrossRef]
11. Pate, R.R.; O'Neill, J.R.; Lobelo, F. The evolving definition of "sedentary". *Exerc. Sport. Sci. Rev.* **2008**, *36*, 173–178. [CrossRef]
12. Tudor-Locke, C.; Washington, T.L.; Ainsworth, B.E.; Troiano, R.P. Linking the American Time Use Survey (ATUS) and the Compendium of Physical Activities: Methods and rationale. *J. Phys. Act. Health* **2009**, *6*, 347–353. [CrossRef]
13. Haskell, W.L.; Lee, I.M.; Pate, R.R.; Powell, K.E.; Blair, S.N.; Franklin, B.A.; Macera, C.A.; Heath, G.W.; Thompson, P.D.; Bauman, A. Physical activity and public health: Updated recommendation for adults from the American College of Sports Medicine and the American Heart Association. *Med. Sci. Sports Exerc.* **2007**, *39*, 1423–1434. [CrossRef]
14. Hirano, T.; Doi, K.; Matsunaga, K.; Takahashi, S.; Donishi, T.; Suga, K.; Oishi, K.; Yasuda, K.; Mimura, Y.; Harada, M.; et al. A Novel Role of Growth Differentiation Factor (GDF)-15 in Overlap with Sedentary Lifestyle and Cognitive Risk in COPD. *J. Clin. Med.* **2020**, *9*, 2737. [CrossRef]
15. Miller, M.R.; Hankinson, J.; Brusasco, V.; Burgos, F.; Casaburi, R.; Coates, A.; Crapo, R.; Enright, P.; van der Grinten, C.P.; Gustafsson, P.; et al. Standardisation of spirometry. *Eur. Respir. J.* **2005**, *26*, 319–338. [CrossRef]
16. Craig, C.L.; Marshall, A.L.; Sjostrom, M.; Bauman, A.E.; Booth, M.L.; Ainsworth, B.E.; Pratt, M.; Ekelund, U.; Yngve, A.; Sallis, J.F.; et al. International physical activity questionnaire: 12-country reliability and validity. *Med. Sci. Sports Exerc.* **2003**, *35*, 1381–1395. [CrossRef] [PubMed]
17. Bull, F.C.; Maslin, T.S.; Armstrong, T. Global physical activity questionnaire (GPAQ): Nine country reliability and validity study. *J. Phys. Act. Health* **2009**, *6*, 790–804. [CrossRef] [PubMed]
18. Ishikawa-Takata, K.; Tabata, I.; Sasaki, S.; Rafamantanantsoa, H.H.; Okazaki, H.; Okubo, H.; Tanaka, S.; Yamamoto, S.; Shirota, T.; Uchida, K.; et al. Physical activity level in healthy free-living Japanese estimated by doubly labelled water method and International Physical Activity Questionnaire. *Eur. J. Clin. Nutr.* **2008**, *62*, 885–891. [CrossRef] [PubMed]
19. Taylor, H.L.; Jacobs, D.R., Jr.; Schucker, B.; Knudsen, J.; Leon, A.S.; Debacker, G. A questionnaire for the assessment of leisure time physical activities. *J. Chronic. Dis.* **1978**, *31*, 741–755. [CrossRef] [PubMed]
20. Baecke, J.A.; Burema, J.; Frijters, J.E. A short questionnaire for the measurement of habitual physical activity in epidemiological studies. *Am. J. Clin. Nutr.* **1982**, *36*, 936–942. [CrossRef] [PubMed]

21. Washburn, R.A.; Smith, K.W.; Jette, A.M.; Janney, C.A. The Physical Activity Scale for the Elderly (PASE): Development and evaluation. *J. Clin. Epidemiol.* **1993**, *46*, 153–162. [CrossRef]
22. Ries, A.L. Impact of chronic obstructive pulmonary disease on quality of life: The role of dyspnea. *Am. J. Med.* **2006**, *119*, 12–20. [CrossRef] [PubMed]
23. Mahler, D.A.; Wells, C.K. Evaluation of clinical methods for rating dyspnea. *Chest* **1988**, *93*, 580–586. [CrossRef]
24. Bestall, J.C.; Paul, E.A.; Garrod, R.; Garnham, R.; Jones, P.W.; Wedzicha, J.A. Usefulness of the Medical Research Council (MRC) dyspnoea scale as a measure of disability in patients with chronic obstructive pulmonary disease. *Thorax* **1999**, *54*, 581–586. [CrossRef] [PubMed]
25. Watz, H.; Waschki, B.; Meyer, T.; Magnussen, H. Physical activity in patients with COPD. *Eur. Respir. J.* **2009**, *33*, 262–272. [CrossRef] [PubMed]
26. Jones, P.W.; Harding, G.; Berry, P.; Wiklund, I.; Chen, W.H.; Kline Leidy, N. Development and first validation of the COPD Assessment Test. *Eur. Respir. J.* **2009**, *34*, 648–654. [CrossRef]
27. Bradley, M.M.; Lang, P.J. Measuring emotion: The Self-Assessment Manikin and the Semantic Differential. *J. Behav. Ther. Exp. Psychiatry* **1994**, *25*, 49–59. [CrossRef]
28. Wolkove, N.; Fu, L.Y.; Purohit, A.; Colacone, A.; Kreisman, H. Meal Induced Oxygen Desaturation and Dyspnea in Chronic Obstructive Pulmonary Disease. *Can. Respir. J.* **1998**, *5*, 347020. [CrossRef]
29. Tangri, S.; Woolf, C.R. The breathing pattern in chronic obstructive lung disease during the performance of some common daily activities. *Chest* **1973**, *63*, 126–127. [CrossRef]
30. Smith, J.; Wolkove, N.; Colacone, A.; Kreisman, H. Coordination of eating, drinking and breathing in adults. *Chest* **1989**, *96*, 578–582. [CrossRef]
31. Martinez, F.J.; Couser, J.I.; Celli, B.R. Respiratory response to arm elevation in patients with chronic airflow obstruction. *Am. Rev. Respir. Dis.* **1991**, *143*, 476–480. [CrossRef]
32. Celli, B.R.; Rassulo, J.; Make, B.J. Dyssynchronous breathing during arm but not leg exercise in patients with chronic airflow obstruction. *N. Engl. J. Med.* **1986**, *314*, 1485–1490. [CrossRef]
33. Lee, L.; Friesen, M.; Lambert, I.R.; Loudon, R.G. Evaluation of dyspnea during physical and speech activities in patients with pulmonary diseases. *Chest* **1998**, *113*, 625–632. [CrossRef] [PubMed]
34. Binazzi, B.; Lanini, B.; Romagnoli, I.; Garuglieri, S.; Stendardi, L.; Bianchi, R.; Gigliotti, F.; Scano, G. Dyspnea during speech in chronic obstructive pulmonary disease patients: Effects of pulmonary rehabilitation. *Respiration* **2011**, *81*, 379–385. [CrossRef]
35. O'Donnell, D.E.; Revill, S.M.; Webb, K.A. Dynamic hyperinflation and exercise intolerance in chronic obstructive pulmonary disease. *Am. J. Respir. Crit. Care Med.* **2001**, *164*, 770–777. [CrossRef]
36. Hirano, T.; Matsunaga, K.; Hamada, K.; Uehara, S.; Suetake, R.; Yamaji, Y.; Oishi, K.; Asami, M.; Edakuni, N.; Ogawa, H.; et al. Combination of assist use of short-acting beta-2 agonists inhalation and guidance based on patient-specific restrictions in daily behavior: Impact on physical activity of Japanese patients with chronic obstructive pulmonary disease. *Respir. Investig.* **2019**, *57*, 133–139. [CrossRef] [PubMed]
37. Shioya, T.; Sato, S.; Iwakura, M.; Takahashi, H.; Terui, Y.; Uemura, S.; Satake, M. Improvement of physical activity in chronic obstructive pulmonary disease by pulmonary rehabilitation and pharmacological treatment. *Respir. Investig.* **2018**, *56*, 292–306. [CrossRef] [PubMed]
38. Perez, T.A.; Castillo, E.G.; Ancochea, J.; Pastor Sanz, M.T.; Almagro, P.; Martinez-Camblor, P.; Miravitlles, M.; Rodriguez-Carballeira, M.; Navarro, A.; Lamprecht, B.; et al. Sex differences between women and men with COPD: A new analysis of the 3CIA study. *Respir. Med.* **2020**, *171*, 106105. [CrossRef]
39. Katsura, H.; Yamada, K.; Wakabayashi, R.; Kida, K. Gender-associated differences in dyspnoea and health-related quality of life in patients with chronic obstructive pulmonary disease. *Respirology* **2007**, *12*, 427–432. [CrossRef]
40. Pitta, F.; Takaki, M.Y.; Oliveira, N.H.; Sant'anna, T.J.; Fontana, A.D.; Kovelis, D.; Camillo, C.A.; Probst, V.S.; Brunetto, A.F. Relationship between pulmonary function and physical activity in daily life in patients with COPD. *Respir. Med.* **2008**, *102*, 1203–1207. [CrossRef]

Disclaimer/Publisher's Note: The statements, opinions and data contained in all publications are solely those of the individual author(s) and contributor(s) and not of MDPI and/or the editor(s). MDPI and/or the editor(s) disclaim responsibility for any injury to people or property resulting from any ideas, methods, instructions or products referred to in the content.

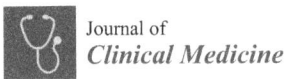

Article

Computed Tomography Lung Density Analysis: An Imaging Biomarker Predicting Physical Inactivity in Chronic Obstructive Pulmonary Disease: A Pilot Study

Yoriyuki Murata [1], Tsunahiko Hirano [1,*], Keiko Doi [1], Ayumi Fukatsu-Chikumoto [1], Kazuki Hamada [1], Keiji Oishi [1], Tomoyuki Kakugawa [2], Masafumi Yano [3] and Kazuto Matsunaga [1]

1. Department of Respiratory Medicine and Infectious Disease, Graduate School of Medicine, Yamaguchi University, Ube 755-8505, Japan; yomurata@yamaguchi-u.ac.jp (Y.M.); decem119@yamaguchi-u.ac.jp (K.D.); chiku05@yamaguchi-u.ac.jp (A.F.-C.); khamada@yamaguchi-u.ac.jp (K.H.); ohishk@yamaguchi-u.ac.jp (K.O.); kazmatsu@yamaguchi-u.ac.jp (K.M.)
2. Department of Pulmonology and Gerontology, Graduate School of Medicine, Yamaguchi University, Ube 755-8505, Japan; kakugawa@yamaguchi-u.ac.jp
3. Department of Medicine and Clinical Science, Graduate School of Medicine, Yamaguchi University, Ube 755-8505, Japan; yanoma@yamaguchi-u.ac.jp
* Correspondence: tsuna@yamaguchi-u.ac.jp; Tel.: +81-836-22-2248

Abstract: Physical inactivity correlates with poor prognosis in chronic obstructive pulmonary disease (COPD) and is suggested to be related to lung hyperinflation. We examined the association between physical activity and the expiratory to inspiratory (E/I) ratio of mean lung density (MLD), the imaging biomarker of resting lung hyperinflation. COPD patients (n = 41) and healthy controls (n = 12) underwent assessment of pulmonary function and physical activity with an accelerometer, as well as computed tomography at full inspiration and expiration. E/I_{MLD} was calculated by measuring inspiratory and expiratory MLD. Exercise (EX) was defined as metabolic equivalents × duration (hours). COPD patients had higher E/I_{MLD} (0.975 vs. 0.964) than healthy subjects. When dividing COPD patients into sedentary (EX < 1.5) and non-sedentary (EX ≥ 1.5) groups, E/I_{MLD} in the sedentary group was statistically higher than that in the non-sedentary group (0.983 vs. 0.972). E/I_{MLD} > 0.980 was a good predictor of sedentary behavior in COPD (sensitivity, 0.815; specificity, 0.714). Multivariate analysis showed that E/I_{MLD} was associated with sedentary behavior (odds ratio, 0.39; $p = 0.04$), independent of age, symptomology, airflow obstruction, and pulmonary diffusion. In conclusion, higher E/I_{MLD} scores are associated with sedentary behavior and can be a useful imaging biomarker for the early detection of physical inactivity in COPD.

Keywords: physical activity; sedentary behavior; density analysis

1. Introduction

Physical activity (PA) in patients with chronic obstructive pulmonary disease (COPD) is lower than that in healthy subjects [1], and this decline is associated with a greater risk of mortality and hospitalization [2–4]. PA in patients with COPD is related to many factors, including age, sex, and the BODE index, which synthesizes information on body mass index, degree of airflow obstruction, dyspnea, and exercise (EX) capacity [5].

PA and EX tolerance in patients with COPD have previously been evaluated using self-administered questionnaires, step counts per day, and evaluations of the 6 min walking distance (6MWD). Of late, triaxial accelerometers have been more sensitive predictors of mortality and hospitalization [3,4]; however, PA evaluation with this method necessitates a dedicated measuring device and reliable measurement data recorded on at least three dry (no rain) weekdays [6]. Therefore, this evaluation method is not practical for all patients with COPD.

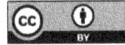

Physical inactivity has been observed even in the early stages of COPD, before the onset of breathlessness [7]. Recently, the usefulness of inspiratory–expiratory computed tomography (CT) has been reported in patients with COPD [8]. Specifically, the expiratory to inspiratory (E/I) ratio of the mean lung density (MLD; E/I_{MLD}), an imaging biomarker, has been reportedly used for the evaluation of small airway disease [9–11]. E/I_{MLD} has been associated with pulmonary function [10–12] and EX tolerance [13]; moreover, it can detect lung hyperinflation, measured as residual volume (RV)/total lung capacity (TLC), more accurately than can the change in relative lung volume, with attenuation values between −860 and −950 Hounsfield units (HU) [14].

In COPD patients, airflow obstruction occurs due to airway wall inflammation and thickening due to inflammatory cell infiltration [15,16]. The resulting air trapping and lung hyperinflation, which are characteristic features of COPD, are more strongly associated with decreased PA than is airflow obstruction [17–19], and reports suggest that these two factors contribute to the vicious cycles of COPD aggravation [20]. If lung hyperinflation is closely associated with the mechanisms of physical inactivity, then E/I_{MLD} may be useful for detecting physical inactivity and predicting poor prognoses in COPD, given that CT is commonly performed for the assessment of patients with COPD.

Therefore, the aim of the present study was to evaluate the association between PA and E/I_{MLD} and to examine the ability of imaging biomarkers to detect physical inactivity in patients with COPD. The hypothesis was that E/I_{MLD} is associated with physical inactivity in COPD. To the best of our knowledge, no prior studies have evaluated this association.

2. Materials and Methods

2.1. Study Design and Subjects

Between 2016 and 2020, ambulatory patients with COPD aged > 40 years at the Yamaguchi University Hospital were recruited for this cross-sectional prospective study. We did not perform power calculations to determine the optimal sample size for statistical significance because this was an exploratory study investigating the association between lung density analysis and PA in a small enrolled sample. We also recruited 12 healthy controls, aged > 40 years, who underwent CT for further evaluation of abnormal findings detected during medical examinations and did not demonstrate any abnormalities on the CT images. All participants underwent pulmonary function tests. COPD was diagnosed according to a post bronchodilator forced expiratory volume in a 1 s/forced vital capacity (FEV_1/FVC) ratio of < 70%. The exclusion criteria were as follows: poor disease control; presence of other diseases that could affect walking, such as lower limb paralysis; requirement of long-term oxygen therapy; and presence of malignant tumors, which can restrict PA. All patients were stable and had not experienced exacerbation for at least 4 weeks. The symptomology was evaluated using the COPD Assessment Test (CAT) and the Modified Medical Research Council (mMRC) Dyspnea Scale. All participants received an explanation of the study and provided written informed consent prior to participation. The study was approved by the institutional review board (No. H27-204-3) of Yamaguchi University Hospital and has been registered in the UMIN Clinical Trials Registry (UMIN 000024749). The protocol was in accordance with the principles of the Declaration of Helsinki and its later amendments.

2.2. PA Evaluations

PA was measured using an accelerometer (Active Style Pro HJA-750C; OMRON HEALTHCARE Co., Ltd., Kyoto, Japan). Although this device is small (30 × 52 × 12 mm) and lightweight (approximately 23 g), it can effectively estimate metabolic equivalents (METs) every 10 s using an internal triaxial accelerometer. All participants wore this device during all waking hours for 2 consecutive weeks. Their PA levels, denoted as EX values, were defined as METs multiplied by their durations (i.e., METs × hour/day) during the last 3 days of monitoring (excluding rainy days and holidays), according to the methodology described in previous studies [6,21]. The duration of each PA with a value of > 1–4 METs was measured in minutes. Patients with COPD showing EX values of < 1.5 (equivalent to < 30 min of walking time per day) and those showing EX values of ≥ 1.5 were divided into the sedentary and non-sedentary groups, respectively [22,23].

2.3. CT Scanning and Lung Density Analysis

All participants underwent volumetric chest CT scans at full inspiration, and expiration was measured using a scanner (Aquilion 64, Toshiba Medical Systems, Otawara, Japan) with the following parameters: 120 kVp; thickness, 1 mm; and rotation time, 0.28–0.5 s. Density analyses were performed using a commercial workstation (Virtual Place; AZE Inc., Tokyo, Japan), as described below. The average HU value for the total lung density area (−1000 to −300 HU) on CT conducted at inspiration was calculated as the inspiratory MLD (I). Expiratory MLD (E) was determined at expiration. E/I_{MLD} was denoted as the E/I ratio [24]. An increase in the E/I ratio, which occurs when there is little difference in HU between inspiration and expiration, indicates the presence of more severe lung hyperinflation and air trapping [9,12,14]. A low attenuation area (LAA) was defined as an area with an attenuation value of < −950 HU in the lung parenchyma.

2.4. Statistical Analyses

All statistical analyses were performed using EZR statistical software (version 1.40; Saitama Medical Center, Jichi Medical University, Shimotsuke, Japan); a modified version of the R commander that was designed to add statistical functions (The R Project for Statistical Computing, Vienna, Austria) [25]. Continuous variables are presented as medians ± interquartile ranges, and categorical variables are presented as numbers and percentages, as appropriate. Comparisons between two continuous variables were performed using the Mann–Whitney U test, whereas those between two categorical variables were performed using Fisher's exact test. Spearman's rank correlation analysis was performed to detect the correlations between E/I_{MLD} and various EX parameters. To identify the predictive factors for sedentary behavior in COPD, we used multivariate logistic regression analysis to calculate adjusted odds ratios (ORs) and the associated 95% confidence intervals (CIs). Variables that reportedly affect PA, including age, CAT score, percent predicted FEV_1 (%FEV_1), and percent predicted carbon monoxide diffusing capacity (%DLCO), were included in the multivariate model [5]. A two-side p-value of < 0.05 was considered statistically significant.

3. Results

3.1. Healthy Subjects vs. Patients with COPD

The baseline characteristics of the participants are shown in Table 1. We enrolled 12 healthy controls and 41 patients with stable COPD. Compared with healthy subjects, patients with COPD were older and had higher CAT scores. Values of pulmonary function parameters such as FEV_1 and FVC were also significantly lower in patients with COPD than in healthy subjects. Among the patients with COPD, 19, 20, and 2 showed stages 1, 2, and 3 COPD, respectively, according to the Global Initiative for Chronic Obstructive Lung Disease (GOLD) criteria. Thus, almost all the enrolled patients presented with mild-to-moderate COPD. COPD patients with mMRC ≥ 2 exhibited worsening airflow obstruction, hyperinflation, and pulmonary diffusion compared with healthy subjects (Table S1). The EX values were significantly lower (median, 2.29 vs. 4.97 METs × hour; $p < 0.0001$), while E/I_{MLD} values were significantly higher (0.975 vs. 0.964, $p = 0.01$) for patients with COPD than for healthy subjects (Figure 1). E/I_{MLD} was significantly correlated with EX for all participants (patients with COPD and healthy subjects: Figure 2, r = −0.36, $p = 0.008$) and for patients with COPD (Table 2, r = −0.32, $p = 0.04$), but not for healthy subjects (Table 2, r = −0.32, $p = 0.32$). Moreover, E/I_{MLD} showed a significant negative correlation with the duration of higher intensity EX (e.g., > 3 METs; Table 2).

Table 1. Clinical characteristics of healthy subjects and patients with COPD.

	HS (n = 12)	COPD (n = 41)	p-Value
Sex (M/F)	6/6	41/0	<0.0001
Age (year)	62 (56–70)	71 (67–74)	0.02
BMI (kg/m^2)	21.4 (19.8–23.8)	22.8 (20.4–24.4)	0.33
Smoking index (pack-year)	10 (0.0–31)	45 (29–103)	0.0004
CAT	4 (3.5–6.3)	11 (7.8–14.5)	0.001
mMRC Dyspnea Scale (0/1/2/3/4)	6/6/0/0/0	17/15/5/3/0	0.62
FEV_1 (L)	2.65 (2.39–3.16)	2.21 (1.90–2.46)	0.002
FEV_1/FVC (%)	78.2 (75.8–86.9)	63.6 (58.0–66.4)	<0.0001
FEV_1 % pred (%)	110 (103–115)	77.0 (65.9–85.6)	<0.0001
GOLD stage (1/2/3/4)	-	19/20/2/0	-
FVC % pred (%)	110 (105–120)	103 (88.6–118)	0.08
RV % pred (%)	114 (103–117)	105 (98.7–128)	0.84
RV/TLC % pred (%)	100 (90.7–113)	90.7 (80.7–102)	0.46
IC/TLC (%)	44.4 (42.5–49.6)	41.4 (34.1–45.8)	0.18
%DLCO (%)	105 (96.8–125)	90.1 (75.8–109)	0.09
%DLCO/VA (%)	94.6 (89.9–105)	75.0 (65.1–102)	0.18

Data are presented as medians (interquartile ranges). Definition of abbreviations: HS, healthy subjects; COPD, chronic obstructive pulmonary disease; BMI, body mass index; CAT, COPD Assessment Test; mMRC, Modified Medical Research Council; GOLD, Global Initiative for Chronic Obstructive Lung Disease; FEV_1, forced expiratory volume in 1 s; FVC, forced vital capacity; RV, residual volume; TLC, total lung capacity; IC, inspiratory capacity; DLCO, carbon monoxide diffusing capacity; VA, alveolar volume.

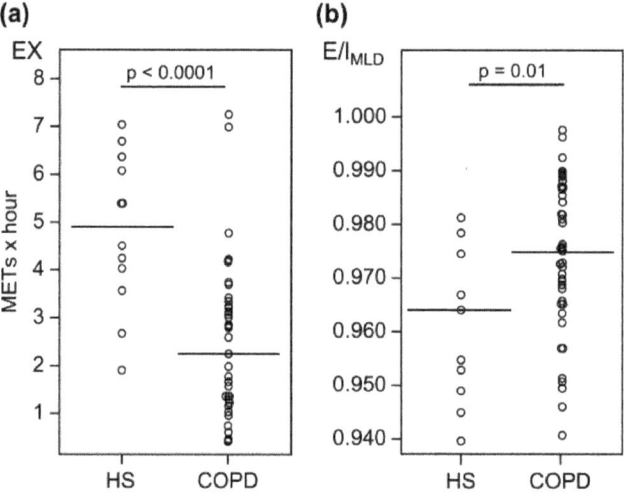

Figure 1. Comparison of EX (a) and E/I$_{MLD}$ (b) values between healthy subjects and patients with COPD. EX values are lower (median, 2.29 vs. 4.97 METs × hour; $p < 0.0001$) (a); while E/I$_{MLD}$ values are higher (median, 0.975 vs. 0.964; $p = 0.01$) for patients with COPD than for healthy subjects (b). Definition of abbreviations: HS, healthy subjects; COPD, chronic obstructive pulmonary disease; METs, metabolic equivalents; EX, exercise (METs × hour); E/I$_{MLD}$, expiratory to inspiratory ratio of the mean lung density. The horizontal bars indicate median values.

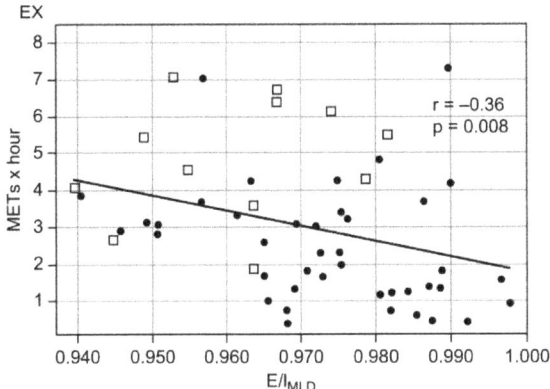

Figure 2. Correlations between EX and E/I$_{MLD}$ values for healthy subjects and patients with COPD. □, healthy subjects; ●, patients with COPD. Definition of abbreviations: COPD, chronic obstructive pulmonary disease; METs, metabolic equivalents; EX, exercise (METs × hour); E/I$_{MLD}$, expiratory to inspiratory ratio of the mean lung density.

Table 2. Coefficients of correlation between exercise intensity and E/I$_{MLD}$ for healthy subjects and patients with COPD.

	E/I$_{MLD}$		
	All Subjects (n = 53)	Healthy (n = 12)	COPD (n = 41)
>1 MET duration (min)	−0.18	−0.02	−0.03
>2 MET duration (min)	−0.21	−0.31	−0.15
>3 MET duration (min)	−0.37 †	−0.31	−0.31 *
>4 MET duration (min)	−0.37 †	−0.46	−0.36 *
Exercise (METs × hour)	−0.36 †	−0.32	−0.32 *

* $p < 0.05$, † $p < 0.01$. Data are presented as correlation coefficients. Definition of abbreviations: HS, healthy subjects; COPD, chronic obstructive pulmonary disease; METs, metabolic equivalents; E/I$_{MLD}$, expiratory to inspiratory ratio of the mean lung density.

3.2. Predictive Factors for Detecting Sedentary Behavior in COPD

Table 3 shows the results of comparisons between the sedentary and nonsedentary groups of COPD patients. E/I$_{MLD}$ was significantly higher in the sedentary group than in the nonsedentary group (0.983 vs. 0.972, $p = 0.02$; Table 3, Figure 3a). However, CAT scores and pulmonary function parameters, including FEV$_1$, FVC, DLCO, and LAA%, were not significantly different between the groups, even after adjustments for age, smoking index, and the mMRC Dyspnea Scale score (Table 3). Moreover, an E/I$_{MLD}$ of > 0.980 exhibited a sensitivity of 0.815 and a specificity of 0.714 (area under the receiver operating characteristic [ROC] curve [AUC] = 0.730) (Figure 3b) for the identification of sedentary patients with COPD, whereas an age of > 71 years yielded a sensitivity of 0.704 and a specificity of 0.786 (AUC = 0.745; 95% CI, 0.568–0.922).

The results of multivariate analysis indicated that E/I$_{MLD}$ was significantly associated with sedentary behavior (EX < 1.5) in patients with COPD, with an adjusted OR of 0.39 (95% CI, 0.16–0.95; $p = 0.04$) when accounting for age, CAT score, predicted %FEV$_1$, and %DLCO (Table 4).

Table 3. Comparison between sedentary and nonsedentary groups of patients with COPD.

	Sedentary Group (n = 14)	Nonsedentary Group (n = 27)	p-Value
Sex (M/F)	14/0	27/0	-
Age (years)	75.5 (72.0–80.8)	68.0 (66.0–72.0)	0.01
BMI (kg/m^2)	24.1 (22.0–24.7)	22.7 (20.4–23.9)	0.42
Smoking index (pack-year)	52.9 (41.3–61.5)	38.0 (22.8–51.5)	0.04
CAT	9.5 (7.0–11.8)	12.0 (9.3–16.0)	0.16
mMRC Dyspnea Scale (0/1/2/3/4)	3/7/4/0/0	14/8/1/3/0	0.02
FEV$_1$/FVC (%)	61.6 (58.1–66.2)	63.7 (58.5–66.8)	0.69
FEV$_1$ % pred (%)	74.4 (58.6–83.8)	80.9 (69.8–90.2)	0.26
GOLD stage (1/2/3/4)	5/9/0/0	14/11/2/0	0.33
FVC % pred (%)	98.0 (80.6–121)	104 (93.3–113)	0.67
RV % pred (%)	115 (103–132)	104 (96.1–121)	0.34
RV/TLC % pred (%)	94.3 (81.2–107)	88.8 (80.7–102)	0.87
IC/TLC (%)	39.0 (33.5–41.8)	44.3 (35.8–47.4)	0.10
%DLCO (%)	92.2 (76.3–109)	89.5 (76.2–109)	0.90
%DLCO/VA (%)	68.0 (60.6–85.8)	85.1 (70.1–107)	0.11
Step per hour	59.1 (49.0–61.5)	64.4 (52.9–73.3)	0.17
6MWD (m)	386 (375–417)	412 (372–459)	0.21
LAA (%)	22.2 (20.9–22.8)	22.5 (20.9–25.6)	0.75
E/I$_{MLD}$	0.983 (0.972–0.987)	0.972 (0.959–0.976)	0.02

Data are presented as medians (IQR, interquartile ranges). Definition of abbreviations: COPD, chronic obstructive pulmonary disease; BMI, body mass index; CAT, COPD Assessment Test; mMRC, Modified Medical Research Council; FEV$_1$, forced expiratory volume in 1 s; FVC, forced vital capacity; RV, residual volume; TLC, total lung capacity; IC, inspiratory capacity; DLCO, carbon monoxide diffusing capacity; VA, alveolar volume; 6MWD, 6-min walking distance; SpO$_2$, peripheral oxygen saturation; MWT, 6-min walking test; LAA, low attenuation area; E/I$_{MLD}$, expiratory to inspiratory ratio of the mean lung density.

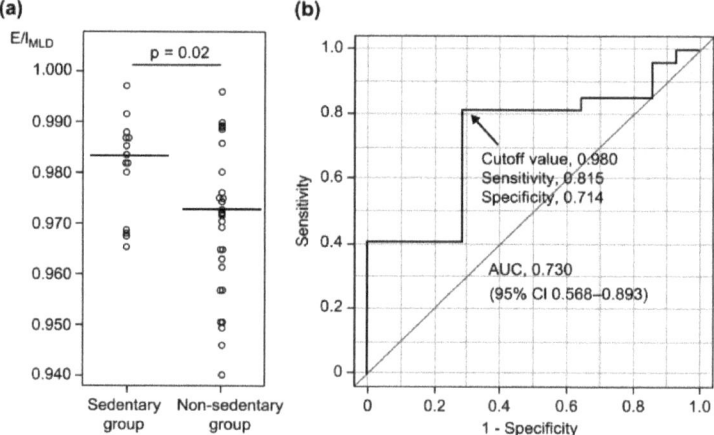

Figure 3. Comparison of E/I$_{MLD}$ for physical activity (**a**) and ROC curve evaluation of the utility of E/I$_{MLD}$ for detecting sedentary behavior in patients with COPD (**b**). A comparison of E/I$_{MLD}$ values between the sedentary (patients with EX values of < 1.5, n = 14) and nonsedentary (patients with EX values of ≥1.5, n = 27) groups demonstrates a statistically significant between-group difference (median, 0.983 vs. 0.972; p = 0.02). The ROC evaluation of the utility of E/I$_{MLD}$ for detecting sedentary behavior in patients with COPD is shown here. If the cutoff value of E/I$_{MLD}$ is 0.980 (arrow), the sensitivity and specificity are 0.815 and 0.714, respectively. The AUC is 0.730 (95% confidence interval, 0.568–0.893). Definition of abbreviations: E/I$_{MLD}$, expiratory to inspiratory ratio of the mean lung density; ROC, receiver operating characteristic; COPD, chronic obstructive pulmonary disease; EX, exercise; AUC, area under the receiver operating characteristic curve. The horizontal bars indicate median values.

Table 4. Univariate and multivariate analyses of factors predicting sedentary behavior in patients with COPD.

Variable	Univariate Analysis		Multivariate Analysis	
	OR (95% CI)	p-Value	OR (95% CI)	p-Value
Age (years)	0.89 (0.80–0.99)	0.03	0.87 (0.75–1.00)	0.05
CAT	1.05 (0.95–1.15)	0.34	1.15 (0.99–1.33)	0.07
FEV$_1$ % pred (%)	1.02 (0.98–1.05)	0.38	1.04 (0.92–1.10)	0.21
%DLCO (%)	1.00 (0.98–1.03)	0.78	0.96 (0.92–1.01)	0.11
E/I$_{MLD}$ (%)	0.47 (0.25–0.87)	0.02	0.39 (0.16–0.95)	0.04

Definition of abbreviations: COPD, chronic obstructive pulmonary disease; OR, odds ratio; CI, confidence interval; CAT, COPD Assessment Test; FEV$_1$, forced expiratory volume in 1 s; DLCO, carbon monoxide diffusing capacity; E/I$_{MLD}$, expiratory to inspiratory ratio of the mean lung density.

4. Discussion

The present study demonstrated that higher E/I$_{MLD}$ values were associated with physical inactivity in stable COPD patients. To the best of our knowledge, this is the first study to demonstrate an association between E/I$_{MLD}$ values and PA in patients with COPD. We also found that a higher E/I$_{MLD}$ value (>0.980) was a predictive factor for physical inactivity in patients with COPD, irrespective of age, symptomology, airflow obstruction, and pulmonary diffusion. These results confirm that higher E/I$_{MLD}$ values, which are associated with air trapping and lung hyperinflation, can be useful for detecting sedentary behavior in patients with COPD. This suggests that E/I$_{MLD}$ can be a new tool for evaluating physical inactivity in patients with COPD (as an alternative to triaxial accelerometers). We showed that E/I$_{MLD}$ evaluated using inspiratory and expiratory CT readings showed a significant negative correlation with PA (Figure 2, Table 2). We also detected sedentary behavior in patients with COPD (Figure 3). In a previous study, E/I$_{MLD}$ was elevated in smokers with predicted FEV$_1$ values of < 80% and/or DLCO values of < 80% [10]. Another study evaluating patients with emphysema showed that E/I$_{MLD}$ was negatively correlated with the predicted %FEV$_1$ in patients with COPD (in contrast to %LAA) [11]. Studies have also shown that E/I$_{MLD}$ values are more strongly associated with air trapping derived from the RV to TLC ratio (RV/TLC) [9,12] and positively correlated with small airway obstruction evaluated by a single-breath nitrogen test [26]. These findings indicate that E/I$_{MLD}$ may be an effective imaging biomarker for detecting air trapping, airflow obstruction, and small airway obstruction in smokers and patients with COPD. This may explain the association between E/I$_{MLD}$ and EX tolerance observed in the previous study [13], as well as the association between E/I$_{MLD}$ and physical inactivity in the present study.

Interestingly, the present study demonstrated that sedentary patients with COPD tended to exhibit mild dyspnea (predominantly mMRC grade 0–1, 71.4%; Table 3). Physical inactivity is highly prevalent, even in patients with COPD who are not aware of severe dyspnea (mMRC grade 0, 45.8%; grade 1, 47.2%) [27], and symptom questionnaires may therefore underestimate physical inactivity in patients with COPD [28]. Similarly, the present study showed that the evaluation of symptoms on the basis of mMRC and CAT scores is not necessarily useful for the earlier detection of physical inactivity in patients with COPD. In addition to the significant negative correlation between E/I$_{MLD}$ and PA in patients with COPD (Figure 2, Table 2), a strong correlation between higher EX intensity and E/I$_{MLD}$ was observed in the present study (r = −0.15 for > 2 METs, −0.31 for > 3 METs, −0.36 for > 4 METs) (Table 2). Minakata et al. reported that PA of higher intensity was reduced in patients with COPD; compared with healthy subjects, patients with COPD showed reductions of 23.1% for ≥ 2.0 METs and 66.9% for ≥ 3.5 METs [29]. This report helps explain why E/I$_{MLD}$ preferentially identifies a decrease in PA of significantly higher intensity.

The PA levels of patients with COPD enrolled in the present study were significantly lower than those of healthy subjects, although the majority of enrolled subjects had mild-to-moderate COPD, and the median predicted FEV$_1$ in patients with COPD was 77.0% (Table 1). Moreover, half the sedentary patients with COPD had GOLD stage 1 COPD

(14/27, 52%; Table 3). Previous studies have shown that FEV_1, inspiratory capacity (IC), RV, and DLCO values are associated with PA in patients with COPD [17–19]. However, our data showed that the values of various pulmonary function parameters, such as airway obstruction (FEV_1), static hyperinflation (IC/TLC), and diffusing capacity (DLCO), were not significantly different between sedentary and nonsedentary patients with COPD (Table 3). These differences may be attributed to the varying backgrounds of the participants. For example, in a previous study that included patients evenly categorized according to GOLD stages 1–4, the mean predicted %FEV_1 was 40–60%, which was significantly lower than that in the present study [17–19]. In other words, prior studies have shown that airway obstruction is associated with physical inactivity in patients with more severe COPD, whereas the present study indicated that E/I_{MLD} is more useful than is spirometry for detecting physical inactivity in patients with less advanced COPD. Further prospective studies are required for a more comprehensive evaluation of the association between PA and lung density.

Of late, CT evaluations have shown that extrapulmonary factors such as skeletal muscles are associated with PA and air trapping [30]. Because E/I_{MLD} is the difference between inspiration and expiration on CT, it may be affected by the strength of the lungs and respiratory muscles. Additional studies should evaluate the association between respiratory muscle volume and density in sedentary patients with COPD in more detail. In the present study, ROC curve analyses indicated that an E/I_{MLD} value of > 0.980 showed good sensitivity with a high AUC value for the detection of sedentary behavior in patients with COPD (Figure 3b). Of course, age was correlated with both physical activity and E/I_{MLD} because age was thought to effect physical activity and progressive hyperinflation in COPD patients. Nevertheless, multivariate analyses showed that the association between E/I_{MLD} and sedentary behavior in patients with COPD was independent of age, CAT score, % predicted FEV_1, and %DLCO (Table 4). Our findings indicate that E/I_{MLD} is useful to screen for physical inactivity prior to symptom progression and onset of lung dysfunction in COPD. Aging was a predictive factor for physical inactivity, but sensitivity was better for E/I_{MLD} than for age. Moreover, the usefulness of bronchodilators for improving PA when evaluating improvements in airway obstruction with COPD has been controversial, as mentioned in a few previous reports [31–38]. In contrast, Takahashi et al. recently reported that tiotropium/olodaterol reduced the duration of PA with 1.0–1.5 METs, thus improving PA [39]. Furthermore, according to the American Thoracic Society guidelines, patients with COPD showing EX intolerance must be treated with long-acting β2-agonist (LABA)/long-acting muscarinic antagonist (LAMA) combination therapy instead of LABA or LAMA monotherapy [40]. This suggests that early detection of physical inactivity may facilitate initial dual bronchodilator treatments to improve PA in inhaler-naive patients with COPD. Other therapeutic interventions, such as long-lasting rehabilitation programs and educational initiatives aimed at increasing PA and thereby optimizing health, also exist [31,41,42]. Moreover, early detection of physical inactivity by the evaluation of E/I_{MLD} may decrease the risk of exacerbation and improve the prognosis of patients with COPD. Although CT increases medical radiation exposure, evaluation of E/I_{MLD} should be considered for patients with COPD who exhibit few symptoms and preserved pulmonary function.

This study has some limitations. First, this was a cross-sectional study conducted at a single institution, and the number of enrolled patients was small. This may have resulted in uncontrolled bias inherent to the study design. Second, most of the targeted patients presented with mild-to-moderate disease, which limits the generalizability of the study findings. Notably, however, the rate of coexistence of severe COPD with heart disease or neuromuscular disorders causing activity restriction is high. Third, certain cardiorespiratory variables that may affect sedentary behavior, such as respiratory muscle force, lung elasticity, and various physiological responses (heart rate, maximal oxygen assumption, and ventilation at maximal EX), could not be accounted for in the present study. Four, all COPD patients were male compared to the female patients in the healthy subjects group (Table 1); therefore, the comparison by sex is not sufficient in this study. The sex differences in COPD patients have been reported to affect dyspnea [43], the severity of CT emphysema [44], and physical inactivity [45]. Future studies should evaluate these topics in a more comprehensive fashion.

5. Conclusions

We demonstrated that higher E/I_{MLD} values were associated with sedentary behavior in patients with mild-to-moderate COPD. The results suggest that this imaging biomarker is a useful tool for the early detection of physical inactivity in patients with COPD, which can improve the quality of life and health trajectories in this patient population. Our findings need to be verified in future highly powered investigations. However, they are expected to guide future study directions and, if confirmed, will ultimately facilitate the development of medical guidelines and interventions.

Supplementary Materials: The following supporting information can be downloaded at: https://www.mdpi.com/article/10.3390/jcm12082959/s1, Table S1. Clinical characteristics of healthy subjects and COPD patients with mMRC grade ≥ 2.

Author Contributions: Conceptualization, Y.M., T.H., T.K., M.Y., and K.M.; methodology, Y.M., T.H., and K.M.; formal analysis, Y.M., K.D., and A.F.-C.; investigation, Y.M., T.H., and K.D.; resources, Y.M., T.H., A.F.-C., K.H., K.O., and K.M.; data curation, Y.M., K.D., and A.F.-C.; writing—original draft preparation, Y.M., T.H., and K.M.; writing—review and editing, Y.M., T.H., and K.M.; project administration, Y.M., T.H., and K.M.; funding acquisition, Y.M., T.H., M.Y., and K.M. All authors have read and agreed to the published version of the manuscript.

Funding: This research was was supported by a grant from the Japan Society for the Promotion of Science (JSPS) KAKENHI (grant number JP21K07675). The funder had no role in the design, conduct, or reporting of this work.

Institutional Review Board Statement: The study was conducted in accordance with the Declaration of Helsinki and approved by the Institutional Review Board of Yamaguchi University Hospital (No. H27-204-3), and it has been registered in the UMIN Clinical Trials Registry (UMIN 000024749).

Informed Consent Statement: Informed consent was obtained from all subjects involved in the study.

Data Availability Statement: The data analyzed during the current study are included in this article. Additional data are available by request to the corresponding author.

Acknowledgments: We thank Hiroe Hotta and Kumiko Teramoto for collecting patient data.

Conflicts of Interest: The authors declare no conflict of interest.

References

1. Pitta, F.; Troosters, T.; Spruit, M.A.; Probst, V.S.; Decramer, M.; Gosselink, R. Characteristics of physical activities in daily life in chronic obstructive pulmonary disease. *Am. J. Respir. Crit. Care Med.* **2005**, *171*, 972–977. [CrossRef] [PubMed]
2. Pitta, F.; Troosters, T.; Probst, V.S.; Spruit, M.A.; Decramer, M.; Gosselink, R. Physical activity and hospitalization for exacerbation of COPD. *Chest* **2006**, *129*, 536–544. [CrossRef] [PubMed]
3. Waschki, B.; Kirsten, A.; Holz, O.; Müller, K.C.; Meyer, T.; Watz, H.; Magnussen, H. Physical activity is the strongest predictor of all-cause mortality in patients with COPD: A prospective cohort study. *Chest* **2011**, *140*, 331–342. [CrossRef]
4. Garcia-Rio, F.; Rojo, B.; Casitas, R.; Lores, V.; Madero, R.; Romero, D.; Galera, R.; Villasante, C. Prognostic value of the objective measurement of daily physical activity in patients with COPD. *Chest* **2012**, *142*, 338–346. [CrossRef] [PubMed]
5. Gimeno-Santos, E.; Frei, A.; Steurer-Stey, C.; de Batlle, J.; Rabinovich, R.A.; Raste, Y.; Hopkinson, N.S.; Polkey, M.I.; van Remoortel, H.; Troosters, T.; et al. Determinants and outcomes of physical activity in patients with COPD: A systematic review. *Thorax* **2014**, *69*, 731–739. [CrossRef]
6. Hirano, T.; Matsunaga, K.; Hamada, K.; Uehara, S.; Suetake, R.; Yamaji, Y.; Oishi, K.; Asami, M.; Edakuni, N.; Ogawa, H.; et al. Combination of assist use of short-acting beta-2 agonists inhalation and guidance based on patient-specific restrictions in daily behaviour: Impact on physical activity of Japanese patients with chronic obstructive pulmonary disease. *Respir. Investig.* **2019**, *57*, 133–139. [CrossRef]
7. Gouzi, F.; Préfaut, C.; Abdellaoui, A.; Vuillemin, A.; Molinari, N.; Ninot, G.; Caris, G.; Hayot, M. Evidence of an early physical activity reduction in chronic obstructive pulmonary disease patients. *Arch. Phys. Med. Rehabil.* **2011**, *92*, 1611–1617.e2. [CrossRef]

8. Gawlitza, J.; Henzler, T.; Trinkmann, F.; Nekolla, E.; Haubenreisser, H.; Brix, G. COPD imaging on a 3rd generation dual-source CT: Acquisition of paired inspiratory-expiratory chest scans at an overall reduced radiation risk. *Diagnostics* **2020**, *10*, 1106. [CrossRef]
9. Eda, S.; Kubo, K.; Fujimoto, K.; Matsuzawa, Y.; Sakai, F. The relations between expiratory chest CT using helical CT and pulmonary function tests in emphysema. *Am. J. Respir. Crit. Care Med.* **1997**, *155*, 1290–1294. [CrossRef]
10. Kubo, K.; Eda, S.; Yamamoto, H.; Fujimoto, K.; Matsuzawa, Y.; Hasegawa, Y.; Sone, S.; Sakai, F. Expiratory and inspiratory chest computed tomography and pulmonary function tests in cigarette smokers. *Eur. Respir. J.* **1999**, *13*, 252–256. [CrossRef]
11. O'Donnell, R.A.; Peebles, C.; Ward, J.A.; Daraker, A.; Angco, G.; Broberg, P.; Pierrou, S.; Lund, J.; Holgate, S.T.; Davies, D.E.; et al. Relationship between peripheral airway dysfunction, airway obstruction, and neutrophilic inflammation in COPD. *Thorax* **2004**, *59*, 837–842. [CrossRef]
12. Mets, O.M.; Murphy, K.; Zanen, P.; Gietema, H.A.; Lammers, J.W.; van Ginneken, B.; Prokop, M.; de Jong, P.A. The relationship between lung function impairment and quantitative computed tomography in chronic obstructive pulmonary disease. *Eur. Radiol.* **2012**, *22*, 120–128. [CrossRef]
13. Hersh, C.P.; Washko, G.R.; Estépar, R.S.J.; Lutz, S.; Friedman, P.J.; Han, M.K.; Hokanson, J.E.; Judy, P.F.; Lynch, D.A.; Make, B.J.; et al. Paired inspiratory-expiratory chest CT scans to assess for small airways disease in COPD. *Respir. Res.* **2013**, *14*, 42. [CrossRef]
14. Mets, O.M.; Zanen, P.; Lammers, J.W.; Isgum, I.; Gietema, H.A.; van Ginneken, B.; Prokop, M.; de Jong, P.A. Early identification of small airways disease on lung cancer screening CT: Comparison of current air trapping measures. *Lung* **2012**, *190*, 629–633. [CrossRef]
15. Hogg, J.C.; Chu, F.; Utokaparch, S.; Woods, R.; Elliott, W.M.; Buzatu, L.; Cherniack, R.M.; Rogers, R.M.; Sciurba, F.C.; Coxson, H.O.; et al. The nature of small-airway obstruction in chronic obstructive pulmonary disease. *N. Engl. J. Med.* **2004**, *24*, 2645–2653. [CrossRef]
16. Hogg, J.C.; Paré, P.D.; Hackett, T.L. The contribution of small airway obstruction to the pathogenesis of chronic obstructive pulmonary disease. *Physiol. Rev.* **2017**, *97*, 529–552. [CrossRef] [PubMed]
17. Garcia-Rio, F.; Lores, V.; Mediano, O.; Rojo, B.; Hernanz, A.; López-Collazo, E.; Alvarez-Sala, R. Daily physical activity in patients with chronic obstructive pulmonary disease is mainly associated with dynamic hyperinflation. *Am. J. Respir. Crit. Care Med.* **2009**, *180*, 506–512. [CrossRef]
18. Lahaije, A.J.; ven Helvoort, H.A.; Dekhuijzen, P.N.; Vercoulen, J.H.; Heijdra, Y.F. Resting and ADL-induced dynamic hyperinflation explain physical inactivity in COPD better than FEV1. *Respir. Med.* **2013**, *107*, 834–840. [CrossRef]
19. Hartman, J.E.; Boezen, H.M.; de Greef, M.H.; Ten Hacken, N.H. Physical and psychosocial factors associated with physical activity in patients with chronic obstructive pulmonary disease. *Arch. Phys. Med. Rehabil.* **2013**, *94*, 2396–2402.e7. [CrossRef]
20. Troosters, T.; van der Molen, T.; Polkey, M.; Rabinovich, R.A.; Vogiatzis, I.; Weisman, I.; Kulich, K. Improving physical activity in COPD: Towards a new paradigm. *Respir. Res.* **2013**, *14*, 115. [CrossRef] [PubMed]
21. Watz, H.; Waschki, B.; Meyer, T.; Magnussen, H. Physical activity in patients with COPD. *Eur. Respir. J.* **2009**, *33*, 262–272. [CrossRef]
22. Haskell, W.L.; Lee, I.M.; Pate, R.R.; Powell, K.E.; Blair, S.N.; Franklin, B.A.; Macera, C.A.; Heath, G.W.; Thompson, P.D.; Bauman, A. Physical activity and public health: Updated recommendation for adults from the American College of Sports Medicine and the American Heart Association. *Circulation* **2007**, *116*, 1081–1093. [CrossRef]
23. Tremblay, M.S.; Aubert, S.; Barnes, J.D.; Saunders, T.J.; Carson, V.; Latimer-Cheung, A.E.; Chastin, S.F.M.; Altenburg, T.M.; Chinapaw, M.J.M. Sedentary Behavior Research Network (SBRN)—Terminology Consensus Project process and outcome. *Int. J. Behav. Nutr. Phys. Act.* **2017**, *14*, 75. [CrossRef] [PubMed]
24. Bodduluri, S.; Reinhardt, J.M.; Hoffman, E.A.; Newell, J.D., Jr.; Nath, H.; Dransfield, M.T.; Bhatt, S.P. Signs of gas trapping in normal lung density Regions in smokers. *Am. J. Respir. Crit. Care Med.* **2017**, *196*, 1404–1410. [CrossRef] [PubMed]
25. Kanda, Y. Investigation of the freely available easy-to-use software 'EZR' for medical statistics. *Bone Marrow Transplant.* **2013**, *48*, 452–458. [CrossRef]
26. Bommart, S.; Marin, G.; Bourdin, A.; Molinari, N.; Klein, F.; Hayot, M.; Vachier, I.; Chanez, P.; Mercier, J.; Vernhet-Kovacsik, H. Relationship between CT air trapping criteria and lung function in small airway impairment quantification. *BMC Pulm. Med.* **2014**, *14*, 29. [CrossRef]
27. Hayata, A.; Minakata, Y.; Matsunaga, K.; Nakanishi, M.; Yamamoto, N. Differences in physical activity according to mMRC grade in patients with COPD. *Int. J. Chronic Obstr. Pulm. Dis.* **2016**, *11*, 2203–2208.
28. van Gestel, A.J.; Clarenbach, C.F.; Stöwhas, A.C.; Rossi, V.A.; Sievi, N.A.; Camen, G.; Russi, E.W.; Kohler, M. Predicting daily physical activity in patients with chronic obstructive pulmonary disease. *PLoS ONE* **2012**, *7*, e48081. [CrossRef]
29. Minakata, Y.; Sugino, A.; Kanda, M.; Ichikawa, T.; Akamatsu, K.; Koarai, A.; Hirano, T.; Nakanishi, M.; Sugiura, H.; Matsunaga, K.; et al. Reduced level of physical activity in Japanese patients with chronic obstructive pulmonary disease. *Respir. Investig.* **2014**, *52*, 41–48. [CrossRef]
30. Hamakawa, Y.; Tanabe, N.; Shima, H.; Terada, K.; Shiraishi, Y.; Maetani, T.; Kubo, T.; Kozawa, S.; Koizumi, K.; Kanezaki, M.; et al. Associations of pulmonary and extrapulmonary computed tomographic manifestations with impaired physical activity in symptomatic patients with chronic obstructive pulmonary disease. *Sci. Rep.* **2022**, *12*, 5608. [CrossRef]

31. Mantoani, L.C.; Rubio, N.; McKinstry, B.; MacNee, W.; Rabinovich, R.A. Interventions to modify physical activity in patients with COPD: A systematic review. *Eur. Respir. J.* **2016**, *48*, 69–81. [CrossRef]
32. O'Donnell, D.E.; Casaburi, R.; Vincken, W.; Puente-Maestu, L.; Swales, J.; Lawrence, D.; Kramer, B. Effect of indacaterol on exercise endurance and lung hyperinflation in COPD. *Respir. Med.* **2011**, *105*, 1030–1036. [CrossRef]
33. Hataji, O.; Naito, M.; Ito, K.; Watanabe, F.; Gabazza, E.C.; Taguchi, O. Indacaterol improves daily physical activity in patients with chronic obstructive pulmonary disease. *Int. J. Chronic Obstr. Pulm. Dis.* **2013**, *8*, 1–5.
34. Troosters, T.; Sciurba, F.C.; Decramer, M.; Siafakas, N.M.; Klioze, S.S.; Sutradhar, S.C.; Weisman, I.M.; Yunis, C. Tiotropium in patients with moderate COPD naive to maintenance therapy: A randomised placebo-controlled trial. *NPJ Prim. Care Respir. Med.* **2014**, *24*, 14003. [CrossRef]
35. Beeh, K.M.; Watz, H.; Puente-Maestu, L.; de Teresa, L.; Jarreta, D.; Caracta, C.; Garcia, G.E.; Magnussen, H. Aclidinium improves exercise endurance, dyspnea, lung hyperinflation, and physical activity in patients with COPD: A randomized, placebo-controlled, crossover trial. *BMC Pulm. Med.* **2014**, *14*, 209. [CrossRef]
36. Nishijima, Y.; Minami, S.; Yamamoto, S.; Ogata, Y.; Koba, T.; Futami, S.; Komuta, K. Influence of indacaterol on daily physical activity in patients with untreated chronic obstructive pulmonary disease. *Int. J. Chronic Obstr. Pulm. Dis.* **2015**, *10*, 439–444.
37. Watz, H.; Mailänder, C.; Baier, M.; Kirsten, A. Effects of indacaterol/glycopyrronium (QVA149) on lung hyperinflation and physical activity in patients with moderate to severe COPD: A randomised, placebo-controlled, crossover study (The MOVE Study). *BMC Pulm. Med.* **2016**, *16*, 95. [CrossRef]
38. Ichinose, M.; Minakata, Y.; Motegi, T.; Ueki, J.; Gon, Y.; Seki, T.; Anzai, T.; Nakamura, S.; Hirata, K. Efficacy of tiotropium/olodaterol on lung volume, exercise capacity, and physical activity. *Int. J. Chronic Obstr. Pulm. Dis.* **2018**, *13*, 1407–1419. [CrossRef]
39. Takahashi, K.; Uchida, M.; Kato, G.; Takamori, A.; Kinoshita, T.; Yoshida, M.; Tajiri, R.; Kojima, K.; Inoue, H.; Kobayashi, H.; et al. First-line treatment with tiotropium/olodaterol improves physical activity in patients with treatment naive chronic obstructive pulmonary disease. *Int. J. Chronic Obstr. Pulm. Dis.* **2020**, *15*, 2115–2126. [CrossRef]
40. Nici, L.; Mammen, M.J.; Charbek, E.; Alexander, P.E.; Au, D.H.; Boyd, C.M.; Criner, G.J.; Donaldson, G.C.; Dreher, M.; Fan, V.S.; et al. Pharmacologic management of chronic obstructive pulmonary disease. An Official American Thoracic Society Clinical Practice Guideline. *Am. J. Respir. Crit. Care Med.* **2020**, *201*, e56–e69. [CrossRef]
41. Pitta, F.; Troosters, T.; Probst, V.S.; Langer, D.; Decramer, M.; Gosselink, R. Are patients with COPD more active after pulmonary rehabilitation? *Chest* **2008**, *134*, 273–280. [CrossRef]
42. Wats, H.; Pitta, F.; Rochester, C.L.; Garcia-Aymerich, J.; ZuWallack, R.; Troosters, T.; Vaes, A.W.; Puhan, M.A.; Jehn, M.; Polkey, M.I.; et al. An official European Respiratory Society statement on physical activity in COPD. *Eur. Repsir. J.* **2014**, *44*, 1521–1537. [CrossRef] [PubMed]
43. Celli, B.; Vestbo, J.; Jenkins, C.R.; Jones, P.W.; Ferguson, G.T.; Calverley, P.M.; Yates, J.C.; Anderson, J.A.; Willits, L.R.; Wise, R.A. Sex differences in mortality and clinical expressions of patients with chronic obstructive pulmonary disease. The TORCH experience. *Am. J. Respir. Crit. Care Med.* **2011**, *183*, 317–322. [CrossRef]
44. Dransfield, M.T.; Washko, G.R.; Foreman, M.G.; Estepar, R.S.; Reilly, J.; Bailey, W.C. Gender differences in the severity of CT emphysema in COPD. *Chest* **2007**, *132*, 464–470. [CrossRef]
45. Sánchez Castillo, S.; Smith, L.; Díaz Suárez, A.; López Sánchez, G.F. Physical activity behaviour in people with COPD residing in Spain: A cross-sectional analysis. *Lung* **2019**, *197*, 769–775. [CrossRef] [PubMed]

Disclaimer/Publisher's Note: The statements, opinions and data contained in all publications are solely those of the individual author(s) and contributor(s) and not of MDPI and/or the editor(s). MDPI and/or the editor(s) disclaim responsibility for any injury to people or property resulting from any ideas, methods, instructions or products referred to in the content.

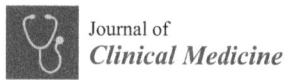

Article

Validation of Simple Prediction Equations for Step Count in Japanese Patients with Chronic Obstructive Pulmonary Disease

Yuichiro Azuma [1], Yoshiaki Minakata [1,*], Mai Kato [1], Masanori Tanaka [2], Yusuke Murakami [1], Seigo Sasaki [1], Kazumi Kawabe [1] and Hideya Ono [1]

[1] Department of Respiratory Medicine, National Hospital Organization Wakayama Hospital, Mihama-cho, Wakayama 644-0044, Japan
[2] Department of Respiratory Medicine, Hashimoto Municipal Hospital, Hashimoto-shi, Wakayama 648-0005, Japan
* Correspondence: minakata.yoshiaki.qy@mail.hosp.go.jp; Tel.: +81-738-22-3256

Abstract: Physical activity is decreased in patients with chronic obstructive pulmonary disease, and decreased physical activity leads to a poor prognosis. To determine an individual's target step count from the measured step counts and predicted step counts, simple and detailed prediction equations for step count were developed. To verify the validity of the simple prediction equation, the validity of the simple equation was evaluated in a different cohort and the correlation between the step counts calculated by the simple equation and those by the detailed prediction equation were evaluated. When the step counts calculated by the simple prediction equation for all participants were compared with the measured step counts, a significant correlation was obtained among them, and the calculated values were found to be reproducible with the measured values in patients with a measured step count of <6500 by Bland–Altman plots. Furthermore, the values calculated by the simple prediction equation and those calculated by the detailed prediction equation showed a significant correlation. In conclusion, the simple prediction equation was considered reasonable.

Keywords: chronic obstructive pulmonary disease; COPD; physical activity; step count; prediction equation

1. Introduction

Physical activity is decreased in patients with chronic obstructive pulmonary disease (COPD) compared to healthy controls [1,2], and decreased physical activity leads to a poor prognosis [3,4]. Physical inactivity is typically associated with all-cause mortality in patients with COPD [5].

Recently, the use of tri-axial accelerometers to evaluate physical activity has attracted attention, and various studies have been conducted [6–14]. However, tri-axial accelerometers are not yet widely available and are not familiar to general physicians. A pedometer is a simple device for evaluating physical activity, and the daily step count has been used as an indicator of physical activity [15–17]. For the general population, the American College of Sports Medicine recommends moderate-intensity cardiorespiratory exercise training for ≥30 min/day ≥5 days/week, vigorous-intensity cardiorespiratory exercise training for ≥20 min/day ≥3 days/week (≥75 min/week), or a combination of moderate- and vigorous-intensity exercise to achieve a total energy expenditure of ≥500–1000 metabolic equivalent (MET)·min/week [18]. However, there have been no recommendations regarding target values of physical activity for patients with COPD. Since patients with COPD have limited physical activity due to reduced lung function, goals comparable to those of healthy individuals may be excessive and should be recommended based on the number of steps expected for each COPD patient.

The factors related to the daily step count among anthropometry, dyspnea, and pulmonary function test findings in Japanese patients with COPD were evaluated and a simple prediction equation for the daily step count using three variables, namely age, a modified Medical Research Council (mMRC) dyspnea scale, and inspiratory capacity (IC), was developed [19]. In addition, since physical activity in COPD patients is considered to be affected by various factors, the use of more factors was examined and a detailed prediction equation for the step count using four variables were developed; these four variables are a 6-min walking distance (6MWD), the mMRC dyspnea scale, the Hospital Anxiety and Depression Scale (consisting of seven items for anxiety; HADS-A) and the forced expiratory volume in one second as a percentage of the predicted value (FEV1 %pred) [20]. Although the detailed prediction equation is considered more accurate, measuring the 6MWD and HADS-A is not easy in daily clinical practice. Therefore, the simple prediction equation may be more practical. Recently, a study has been started to try to increase the step count to reach the target value, which was determined from the measured step counts and predicted values of the step counts by the simple prediction equation [21]. It is necessary to verify whether the simple prediction equation is indeed accurate.

In the current study, to verify the validity of the simple prediction equation, the validity of the simple equation was evaluated in a different cohort and the correlation between the step count calculated by the simple equation and that by the detailed prediction equation was examined.

2. Materials and Methods

2.1. Design

The previous data from a multicenter, prospective cross-sectional study conducted at 23 institutions belonging to National Hospital Organization of Japan were used as secondary use, in which the detailed prediction equation of physical activity in Japanese patients with COPD was developed [20].

2.2. Evaluations

To verify the simple prediction equation of step count for the current cohort, the standard value of the step count for each patient by applying the simple equation was calculated and compared with the actual measured value. Moreover, the step counts calculated by the simple prediction equation was compared with those calculated by the detailed prediction equation and the correlation between the two was examined.

2.3. Measurement of Step Count

Subjects wore a tri-axial accelerometer (Active style Pro HJA-750C [HJA]; Omron Healthcare, Kyoto, Japan) on their waist for 15 to 29 days. From the measured days, the first and last days, rainy days, holidays, days with an average temperature of less than 2.5 °C, days with unusual activities, and days with <8 h per day of measurement time were excluded. Of the remaining valid days, the average of the data from the first three days was used.

2.4. Prediction Equations

The equation by Nakanishi et al. was employed as a simple prediction equation [19]. This is the equation created using a multiple regression analysis with the age, gender, body mass index (BMI), smoking history, IC, forced vital capacity as a percentage of the predicted value (FVC %pred), FEV1 %pred, and mMRC dyspnea scale as independent variables. The simple equation was as follows:

$$\text{step count} = (-0.079 \times \text{age} - 1.595 \times \text{mMRC dyspnea scale} + 2.078 \times \text{IC} + 18.149)^3$$

The equation by Minakata et al. was used as a detailed prediction equation [20]. This is the equation created based on a multiple regression analysis with the age, gender, height, weight, BMI, smoking history, IC, FVC %pred, FEV1/FVC, FEV1 %pred, 6MWD, lowest percutaneous oxygen saturation during the 6MW test, upper arm circumference, subcutaneous fat thickness of triceps branch, grip strength, fasting blood glucose, hemoglobin A1c, red blood cells, hemoglobin, brain natriuretic peptide, albumin, HADS-A, mMRC dyspnea scale, treatment history, rehabilitation history, and comorbidities as independent variables. The detailed equation was as follows:

$$\text{step count} = (0.01 \times 6MWD - 0.666 \times \text{mMRC dyspnea scale} + 0.155 \times \text{HADS-A} + 0.029 \times \text{FEV1 \%pred} + 9.843)^3$$

2.5. Statistical Analyses

Statistical analyses were performed using the GraphPad Prism 7 software program (GraphPad Software, San Diego, CA, USA). Correlation coefficients and Bland–Altman plots were used to compare the measured and calculated step counts. The level of statistical significance was considered to be $p < 0.05$.

2.6. Ethical Consideration

This study was conducted in accordance with the Declaration of Helsinki and was approved by the local ethics committee (IRB Committee of National Hospital Organization Wakayama Hospital; approval number: 03-4; approval date: 22 April 2021) and has been registered with the University Hospital Medical Information Network (UMIN 000047281, 26 March 2022). The contents of this study and the opportunity to reject the agreement were explained on the website of the National Hospital Organization Wakayama Hospital.

3. Results

In all, 253 patients were recruited, and 239 were enrolled. Among enrolled patients, 12 had fewer than 3 valid days, so 227 patients were ultimately included in the analysis (Figure 1). The age was 73.1 ± 6.7 years old, the FEV1 %pred was 62.7% ± 20.9%, and the FVC %pred was 99.6% ± 19.5% (Table 1). Histograms for the indicators used in the prediction equations (6MWD, HADs anxiety score, IC, mMRC dyspnea scale, FEV1 %pred and age) are shown in Figure 2.

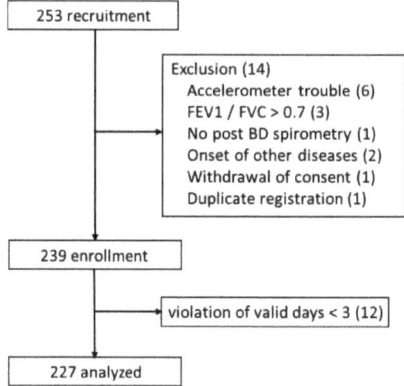

Figure 1. CONSORT diagram. Abbreviations: FEV1, forced expiratory volume in one second; FVC, forced vital capacity; BD, bronchodilator.

Table 1. Patient characteristics.

Gender (Male/Female)	213/14
Age	73.1 ± 6.7
Smoking (pack-year)	64.2 ± 66.5
BMI	22.5 ± 3.4
COPD stage (1/2/3/4)	54/110/48/15
mMRC (0/1/2/3/4)	51/108/42/24/2
IC (L)	2.22 ± 0.56
FVC (L)	3.28 ± 0.78
FVC %pred (%)	99.6 ± 19.5
FEV1 (L)	1.64 ± 0.60
FEV1 %pred (%)	62.7 ± 20.9
FEV1/FVC (%)	49.7 ± 13.2
HADS anxiety score	3.3 ± 2.6
HADS depression score	4.3 ± 3.1

Abbreviations: BMI, body mass index; mMRC, modified British Medical Research Council; IC, inspiratory capacity; FVC, forced vital capacity; FVC %pred, FVC % of predicted; FEV1, forced expiratory volume in one second; FEV1 %pred, FEV1 % of predicted; HADS, Hospital Anxiety and Depression Scale; COPD, chronic obstructive pulmonary disease.

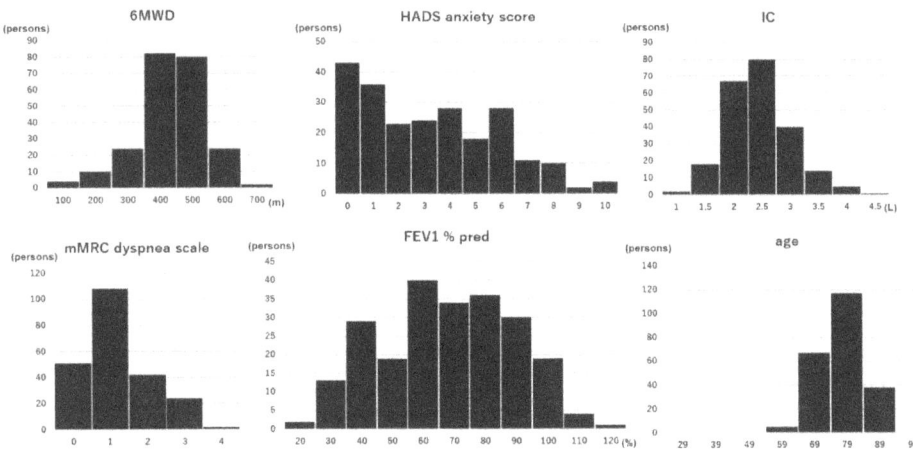

Figure 2. Histograms of the indicators. Abbreviations: 6MWD, 6 min walking distance; HADS, Hospital Anxiety and Depression Scale; IC, inspiratory capacity; mMRC, modified British Medical Research Council; FEV1 %pred, forced expiratory volume in one second % of predicted.

When the step counts calculated by the simple prediction equation for all 227 participants were compared with the measured step counts, a significant correlation was obtained among them (r = 0.344, $p < 0.0001$) (Figure 3A). However, when both step counts were examined with the Bland–Altman plots, there was no fixed bias, although a proportional bias was noted (Figure 3B). According to Nakanishi's report, the values calculated by the simple prediction equation were reproducible with the values measured by the Bland–Altman plots in patients whose measured step count was <6500 steps [19]. In the current population, the calculated values by the simple prediction were also found to be reproducible with the measured values in patients with a measured step count <6500 (Figure 4). Furthermore, reproducibility was obtained in patients with a measured step count <7500.

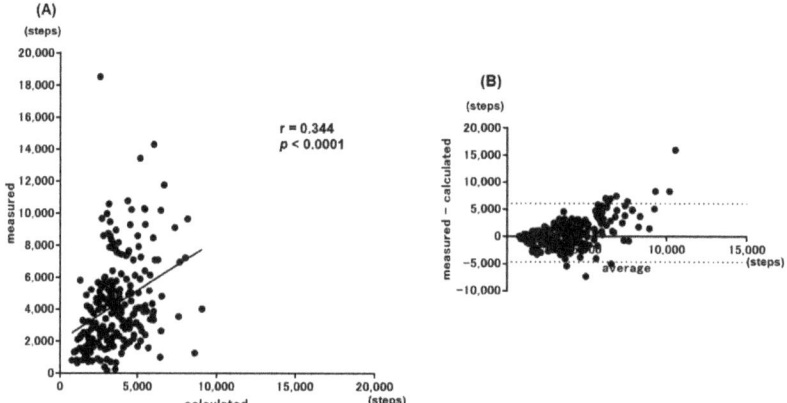

Figure 3. Correlations between the measured values and calculated values by the simple equation. (**A**) Scatter plot and (**B**) Bland–Altman plot.

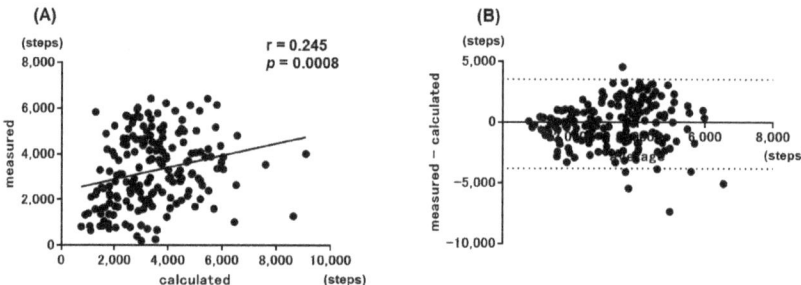

Figure 4. Correlations between the measured values and calculated values by the simple equation in patients with <6500 measured step. (**A**) Scatter plot and (**B**) Bland–Altman plot.

The values calculated by Nakanishi's simple prediction equation and those calculated by Minakata's detailed prediction equation showed a significant correlation (r = 0.657, $p < 0.0001$) (Figure 5).

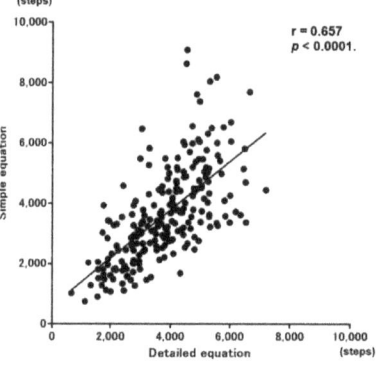

Figure 5. Correlation between the step count calculated by the simple prediction equation and that calculated by the detailed prediction equation.

4. Discussion

The calculated step counts obtained from Nakanishi's simple prediction equation showed a significant correlation with the measured step counts in the current population among patients with a measured step count <6500, confirming its reproducibility. In addition, it showed a significant correlation with the calculated step counts obtained from Minakata's detailed prediction equation.

The simple prediction equation was confirmed to be reliable in patients with COPD and a low step count. The number of patients with a step count <6500 was 185 among 227 recruited patients (81.5%) in the current cohort and 121 among the 162 (74.7%) in the cohort for the development of Nakanishi's simple prediction equation [19]. In the previous meta-analysis on the step counts in patients with COPD, the mean step count was 4579.3 (95% confidence interval 4310.2–5208.4) [22], which suggests that the daily step count of most patients with COPD is <6500. Therefore, Nakanishi's prediction equation was found to be reproducible in different cohorts and may be a useful tool for evaluating the individual predictive step counts in most patients with COPD.

The step counts calculated by the simple prediction equation correlated with those calculated by the detailed prediction equation. The simple equation consisted of the age, mMRC dyspnea scale, and IC, whereas the detailed equation consisted of the 6MWD, mMRC dyspnea scale, HADS-A, and FEV1 %pred. The mMRC dyspnea scale was the only common variable between these two equations. The mMRC dyspnea scale has been reported to correlate with the step count and physical activity in many reports [15,23,24] and detailed prediction equations, and it was considered to be an important factor for the step count. Exercise capacity may be related to physical activity [1,2,25–28], and the 6MWD was included in the detailed equation. However, it was not included in the simple equation because exercise capacity was not evaluated as an independent variable for that equation. Exercise capacity has been reported to be more closely related to IC than to FEV1 %pred [29]. In the current cohort, the 6MWD was multicollinear with IC (r = 0.270, $p < 0.001$), as was FEV1 %pred (r = 0.458, $p < 0.001$) [20]. A decrease in the 6MWD can be predicted by a decrease in the IC/TLC ratio, with a 0.1-unit decrease in the baseline IC/TLC ratio resulting in a 12.7-m decrease in the 6MWD per year [30]. In addition, IC reflects the resting hyperinflation of the lung, and both resting and dynamic hyperinflation contribute to reduced physical activity in COPD [31], which suggests that a lower IC may lead to lower physical activity levels. The 6MWD and FEV1 %pred may thus be able to predict the step count relatively accurately, but IC might be used to some extent instead of them. Although the detailed equation is based on a larger number of variables and seems to be more accurate, the simple equation is easier to use in daily clinical practice.

The attempt to develop a method for setting individual target values of step counts based on the standardized values calculated by the simple prediction equation and the actual measured values is being made. A pilot study in which target values were provided showed the potential to increase the target achievement rate and step count when supplying such values [21]. The efficacy of providing a target value for the step count needs to be verified in future studies with a larger scale.

Limitations

Several limitations associated with the present study warrant mention. First, most of the enrolled patients were men (93.8%). This distribution may be due to the fact that the rate of men with COPD is higher in Japan than in Western countries [32–35], and patients with bronchial asthma, which is thought to be relatively common in women, were excluded from the current cohort. While the number of women was small, gender was included in the regression analysis as an independent variable in both the simple and detailed prediction equations and was not extracted as a factor related to the step count. Further studies including a cohort in which more women participate might be required. Second, there might have been other step-related factors that were not employed as independent variables for the prediction equations. Ichinose et al. reported that the job status (employment) as well as mMRC dyspnea scale were factors related to the step count [24]. Further studies on other influencing factors not used in the current study should thus be conducted. Third, both the simple and detailed prediction equations were based on the Japanese population. Individual studies may be necessary for populations of other countries.

5. Conclusions

The simple equation for predicting the step count of Japanese patients with COPD was validated in different cohorts, and the values calculated by it were significantly correlated with those determined by the detailed prediction equation. The simple prediction equation was considered reasonable.

Author Contributions: Conceptualization, Y.A. and Y.M. (Yoshiaki Minakata); methodology, Y.A.; validation, Y.A. and Y.M. (Yoshiaki Minakata); formal analysis, Y.A.; investigation, Y.A. and Y.M. (Yoshiaki Minakata); resources, Y.A., Y.M. (Yoshiaki Minakata), M.K., M.T., Y.M. (Yusuke Murakami), S.S., K.K. and H.O.; data curation, Y.A.; writing—original draft preparation, Y.A.; writing—review and editing, Y.A., Y.M. (Yoshiaki Minakata), M.K., M.T., Y.M. (Yusuke Murakami), S.S., K.K. and H.O.; visualization, Y.A.; supervision, Y.M. (Yoshiaki Minakata); project administration, Y.A. and Y.M. (Yoshiaki Minakata); funding acquisition, Y.M. (Yoshiaki Minakata). All authors have read and agreed to the published version of the manuscript.

Funding: This research was funded by the Environmental Restoration and Conservation Agency of Japan. URL: http://www.erca.go.jp/erca/english/index.html (accessed on 20 July 2022) [36].

Institutional Review Board Statement: The study was conducted in accordance with the Declaration of Helsinki and approved by the local ethics committee (IRB Committee of National Hospital Organization Wakayama Hospital; approval number: 03-4; approval date: 22 April 2021).

Informed Consent Statement: The contents of this study and the opportunity to reject the agreement were explained on the website of the National Hospital Organization Wakayama Hospital. URL: http://wakayama.hosp.go.jp (accessed on 20 July 2022).

Data Availability Statement: The data that support the findings of this study are available from the corresponding author upon reasonable request.

Acknowledgments: The authors thank Brian Quinn for reading the manuscript.

Conflicts of Interest: The authors declare no conflict of interest.

References

1. Pitta, F.; Troosters, T.; Spruit, M.A.; Probst, V.S.; Decramer, M.; Gosselink, R. Characteristics of physical activities in daily life in chronic obstructive pulmonary disease. *Am. J. Respir. Crit. Care Med.* **2005**, *171*, 972–977. [CrossRef] [PubMed]
2. Minakata, Y.; Sugino, A.; Kanda, M.; Ichikawa, T.; Akamatsu, K.; Koarai, A.; Hirano, T.; Nakanishi, M.; Sugiura, H.; Matsunaga, K.; et al. Reduced level of physical activity in Japanese patients with chronic obstructive pulmonary disease. *Respir. Investig.* **2014**, *52*, 41–48. [CrossRef] [PubMed]
3. Garcia-Aymerich, J.; Lange, P.; Benet, M.; Schnohr, P.; Antó, J.M. Regular physical activity reduces hospital admission and mortality in chronic obstructive pulmonary disease: A population based cohort study. *Thorax* **2006**, *61*, 772–778. [CrossRef] [PubMed]
4. Garcia-Rio, F.; Rojo, B.; Casitas, R.; Lores, V.; Madero, R.; Romero, D.; Galera, R.; Villasante, C. Prognostic value of the objective measurement of daily physical activity in patients with COPD. *Chest* **2012**, *142*, 338–346. [CrossRef]
5. Waschki, B.; Kirsten, A.; Holz, O.; Müller, K.; Meyer, T.; Watz, H.; Magnussen, H. Physical activity is the strongest predictor of all-cause mortality in patients with COPD: A prospective cohort study. *Chest* **2011**, *140*, 331–342. [CrossRef]
6. Furlanetto, K.C.; Donária, L.; Schneider, L.P.; Lopes, J.R.; Ribeiro, M.; Fernandes, K.B.; Hernandes, N.A.; Pitta, F. Sedentary Behavior Is an Independent Predictor of Mortality in Subjects With COPD. *Respir. Care* **2017**, *62*, 579–587. [CrossRef]
7. Cavalheri, V.; Straker, L.; Gucciardi, D.F.; Gardiner, P.A.; Hill, K. Changing physical activity and sedentary behaviour in people with COPD. *Respirology* **2016**, *21*, 419–426. [CrossRef]
8. Geidl, W.; Carl, J.; Cassar, S.; Lehbert, N.; Mino, E.; Wittmann, M.; Wagner, R.; Schultz, K.; Pfeifer, K. Physical Activity and Sedentary Behaviour Patterns in 326 Persons with COPD before Starting a Pulmonary Rehabilitation: A Cluster Analysis. *J. Clin. Med.* **2019**, *8*, 1346. [CrossRef]
9. Wshah, A.; Selzler, A.M.; Hill, K.; Brooks, D.; Goldstein, R. Determinants of Sedentary Behaviour in Individuals with COPD: A Qualitative Exploration Guided by the Theoretical Domains Framework. *COPD J. Chronic Obstr. Pulm. Dis.* **2020**, *17*, 65–73. [CrossRef]

10. Lewthwaite, H.; Effing, T.W.; Lenferink, A.; Olds, T.; Williams, M.T. Improving physical activity, sedentary behaviour and sleep in COPD: Perspectives of people with COPD and experts via a Delphi approach. *PeerJ* **2018**, *6*, e4604. [CrossRef]
11. Bernard, P.; Hains-Monfette, G.; Atoui, S.; Moullec, G. Daily Objective Physical Activity and Sedentary Time in Adults with COPD Using Spirometry Data from Canadian Measures Health Survey. *Can. Respir. J.* **2018**, *2018*, 9107435. [CrossRef]
12. McKeough, Z.J.; Large, S.L.; Spencer, L.M.; Ceng, S.W.M.; McNamara, R.J. An observational study of self-reported sedentary behaviour in people with chronic obstructive pulmonary disease and bronchiectasis. *Braz. J. Phys. Ther.* **2020**, *24*, 399–406. [CrossRef] [PubMed]
13. Alyami, M.M.; Jenkins, S.C.; Hill, K. Walking-based activity and sedentary behavior in Saudi males with chronic obstructive pulmonary disease. *Saudi Med. J.* **2018**, *39*, 506–513. [CrossRef] [PubMed]
14. Hill, K.; Gardiner, P.A.; Cavalheri, V.; Jenkins, S.C.; Healy, G.N. Physical activity and sedentary behaviour: Applying lessons to chronic obstructive pulmonary disease. *Intern. Med. J.* **2015**, *45*, 474–482. [CrossRef]
15. Moy, M.L.; Danilack, V.A.; Weston, N.A.; Garshick, E. Daily step counts in a US cohort with COPD. *Respir. Med.* **2012**, *106*, 962–969. [CrossRef] [PubMed]
16. Danilack, V.A.; Weston, N.A.; Richardson, C.R.; Mori, D.L.; Moy, M.L. Reasons persons with COPD do not walk and relationship with daily step count. *COPD J. Chronic Obstr. Pulm. Dis.* **2014**, *11*, 290–299. [CrossRef]
17. Robinson, S.A.; Cooper, J.A., Jr.; Goldstein, R.L.; Polak, M.; Cruz Rivera, P.N.; Gagnon, D.R.; Samuelson, A.; Moore, S.; Kadri, R.; Richardson, C.R.; et al. A randomised trial of a web-based physical activity self-management intervention in COPD. *ERJ Open Res.* **2021**, *7*, 00158–02021. [CrossRef]
18. Garber, C.E.; Blissmer, B.; Deschenes, M.R.; Franklin, B.A.; Lamonte, M.J.; Lee, I.-M.; Nieman, D.C.; Swain, D.P. American College of Sports Medicine position stand. Quantity and quality of exercise for developing and maintaining cardiorespiratory, musculoskeletal, and neuromotor fitness in apparently healthy adults: Guidance for prescribing exercise. *Med. Sci. Sports Exerc.* **2011**, *43*, 1334–1359. [CrossRef]
19. Nakanishi, M.; Minakata, Y.; Tanaka, R.; Sugiura, H.; Kuroda, H.; Yoshida, M.; Yamamoto, N. Simple standard equation for daily step count in Japanese patients with chronic obstructive pulmonary disease. *Int. J. Chronic Obstr. Pulm. Dis.* **2019**, *14*, 1967–1977. [CrossRef]
20. Minakata, Y.; Sasaki, S.; Azuma, Y.; Kawabe, K.; Ono, H. Reference Equations for Assessing the Physical Activity of Japanese Patients with Chronic Obstructive Pulmonary Disease. *Int. J. Chronic Obstr. Pulm. Dis.* **2021**, *16*, 3041–3053. [CrossRef]
21. Sasaki, S.; Minakata, Y.; Azuma, Y.; Kaki, T.; Kawabe, K.; Ono, H. Effects of individualized target setting on step count in Japanese patients with chronic obstructive pulmonary disease: A pilot study. *Adv. Respir. Med.* **2022**, *90*, 1–8. [CrossRef] [PubMed]
22. Saunders, T.; Campbell, N.; Jason, T.; Dechman, G.; Hernandez, P.; Thompson, K.; Blanchard, C.M. Objectively Measured Steps/Day in Patients with Chronic Obstructive Pulmonary Disease: A Systematic Review and Meta-Analysis. *J. Phys. Act. Health* **2016**, *13*, 1275–1283. [PubMed]
23. Kawagoshi, A.; Kiyokawa, N.; Sugawara, K.; Takahashi, H.; Sakata, S.; Miura, S.; Sawamura, S.; Satake, M. Quantitative assessment of walking time and postural change in patients with COPD using a new triaxial accelerometer system. *Int. J. Chronic Obstr. Pulm. Dis.* **2013**, *8*, 397–404. [CrossRef] [PubMed]
24. Ichinose, M.; Minakata, Y.; Motegi, T.; Takahashi, T.; Seki, M.; Sugaya, S.; Hayashi, N.; Kuwahira, I. A Non-Interventional, Cross-Sectional Study to Evaluate Factors Relating to Daily Step Counts and Physical Activity in Japanese Patients with Chronic Obstructive Pulmonary Disease: STEP COPD. *Int. J. Chronic Obstr. Pulm. Dis.* **2020**, *15*, 3385–3396. [CrossRef] [PubMed]
25. Waschki, B.; Spruit, M.A.; Watz, H.; Albert, P.S.; Shrikrishna, D.; Groenen, M.; Smith, C.; Man, W.D.; Tal-Singer, R.; Edwards, L.D.; et al. Physical activity monitoring in COPD: Compliance and associations with clinical characteristics in a multicenter study. *Respir. Med.* **2012**, *106*, 522–530. [CrossRef]
26. Steele, B.A.; Daniel, T.M. Evaluation of the potential role of serodiagnosis of tuberculosis in a clinic in Bolivia by decision analysis. *Am. Rev. Respir. Dis.* **1991**, *143*, 713–716. [CrossRef]
27. Watz, H.; Waschki, B.; Meyer, T.; Magnussen, H. Physical activity in patients with COPD. *Eur. Respir. J.* **2009**, *33*, 262–272. [CrossRef]
28. Van Remoortel, H.; Hornikx, M.; Demeyer, H.; Langer, D.; Burtin, C.; Decramer, M.; Gosselink, R.; Janssens, W.; Troosters, T. Daily physical activity in subjects with newly diagnosed COPD. *Thorax* **2013**, *68*, 962–963. [CrossRef]
29. O'Donnell, D.E.; Revill, S.M.; Webb, K.A. Dynamic hyperinflation and exercise intolerance in chronic obstructive pulmonary disease. *Am. J. Respir. Crit. Care Med.* **2001**, *164*, 770–777. [CrossRef]
30. Aalstad, L.T.; Hardie, J.A.; Espehaug, B.; Thorsen, E.; Bakke, P.S.; Eagan, T.M.; Frisk, B. Lung hyperinflation and functional exercise capacity in patients with COPD—A three-year longitudinal study. *BMC Pulm. Med.* **2018**, *18*, 187.
31. Lahaije, A.J.; van Helvoort, H.A.; Dekhuijzen, P.N.; Vercoulen, J.H.; Heijdra, Y.F. Resting and ADL-induced dynamic hyperinflation explain physical inactivity in COPD better than FEV1. *Respir. Med.* **2013**, *107*, 834–840. [CrossRef] [PubMed]
32. Ishii, T.; Nishimura, M.; Akimoto, A.; James, M.H.; Jones, P. Understanding low COPD exacerbation rates in Japan: A review and comparison with other countries. *Int. J. Chronic Obstr. Pulm. Dis.* **2018**, *13*, 3459–3471. [CrossRef] [PubMed]
33. Rabe, K.F.; Martinez, F.J.; Ferguson, G.T.; Wang, C.; Singh, D.; Wedzicha, J.A.; Trivedi, R.; Rose, E.S.; Ballal, S.; McLaren, J.; et al. Triple Inhaled Therapy at Two Glucocorticoid Doses in Moderate-to-Very-Severe COPD. *N. Engl. J. Med.* **2020**, *383*, 35–48. [CrossRef] [PubMed]

34. Jiménez, D.; Agustí, A.; Tabernero, E.; Jara-Palomares, L.; Hernando, A.; Ruiz-Artacho, P.; Pérez-Peñate, G.; Rivas-Guerrero, A.; Rodríguez-Nieto, M.J.; Ballaz, A.; et al. Effect of a Pulmonary Embolism Diagnostic Strategy on Clinical Outcomes in Patients Hospitalized for COPD Exacerbation: A Randomized Clinical Trial. *JAMA* **2021**, *326*, 1277–1285. [CrossRef]
35. Vestbo, J.; Anderson, J.A.; Brook, R.D.; Calverley, P.M.; Celli, B.R.; Crim, C.; Martinez, F.; Yates, J.; Newby, D.E.; SUMMIT Investigators. Fluticasone furoate and vilanterol and survival in chronic obstructive pulmonary disease with heightened cardiovascular risk (SUMMIT): A double-blind randomised controlled trial. *Lancet* **2016**, *387*, 1817–1826. [CrossRef]
36. Environmental Restoration and Conservation Agency of Japan. Available online: http://www.erca.go.jp/erca/english/index.html (accessed on 20 July 2022).

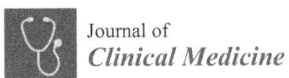

Article

Enhancing Cognition in Older Adults with Mild Cognitive Impairment through High-Intensity Functional Training: A Single-Blind Randomized Controlled Trial

Yulieth Rivas-Campo [1], Agustín Aibar-Almazán [2,*], Carlos Rodríguez-López [3], Diego Fernando Afanador-Restrepo [4], Patricia Alexandra García-Garro [5], Yolanda Castellote-Caballero [2], Alexander Achalandabaso-Ochoa [2] and Fidel Hita-Contreras [2]

[1] Faculty of Human and Social Sciences, University of San Buenaventura-Cali, Santiago de Cali 760016, Colombia; yrivasc@usbcali.edu.co
[2] Department of Health Sciences, Faculty of Health Sciences, University of Jaén, 23071 Jaén, Spain; mycastel@ujaen.es (Y.C.-C.); aaochoa@ujaen.es (A.A.-O.); fhita@ujaen.es (F.H.-C.)
[3] Lecturer University Schools Gimbernat, University of Cantabria, 39005 Santander, Spain; carlinhosdin@gmail.com
[4] Faculty of Health Sciences and Sport, University Foundation of the Área Andina–Pereira, Pereira 660004, Colombia; dafanador4@areandina.edu.co
[5] Faculty of Distance and Virtual Education, Antonio José Camacho University Institution, Santiago de Cali 760016, Colombia; palexandragar-cia@admon.uniajc.edu.co
* Correspondence: aaibar@ujaen.es

Abstract: Physical exercise is a very promising non-pharmacological approach to prevent or reduce the cognitive decline that occurs in people aged 60 years or older. The objective of this study was to determine the effect of a high-intensity intervallic functional training (HIFT) program on cognitive functions in an elderly Colombian population with mild cognitive impairment. A controlled clinical trial was developed with a sample of 132 men and women aged >65 years, linked to geriatric care institutions, which were systematically blind randomized. The intervention group (IG) received a 3-month HIFT program ($n = 64$) and the control group (CG) ($n = 68$) received general physical activity recommendations and practiced manual activities. The outcome variables addressed cognition (MoCA), attention (TMTA), executive functions (TMTB), verbal fluency (VFAT test), processing speed (Digit Symbol Substitution Test-DSST), selective attention and concentration (d2 test). After the analysis, improvement was found in the IG with significant differences with respect to the CG in the level of cognitive impairment (MoCA), attention (TMTA), verbal fluency and concentration ($p < 0.001$). Executive functions (TMTB) showed differences in both groups, being slightly higher in the IG ($p = 0.037$). However, no statistically significant results were found for selective attention ($p = 0.55$) or processing speed ($p = 0.24$). The multiple analysis of covariance (MANCOVA) showed the influence of the education level on all cognition assessments ($p = 0.026$); when adjusting for sociodemographic variables, the influence of the intervention remained significant ($p < 0.001$). This study empirically validates that the implementation of a HIFT program has a positive effect on cognitive functions in elderly people with mild cognitive impairment. Therefore, professionals specialized in the care of this population could consider including functional training programs as an essential part of their therapeutic approaches. The distinctive features of this program, such as its emphasis on functional training and high intensity, appear to be relevant for stimulating cognitive health in the geriatric population.

Keywords: cognition; physical activity; verbal fluency; processing speed; mild cognitive impairment

Citation: Rivas-Campo, Y.; Aibar-Almazán, A.; Rodríguez-López, C.; Afanador-Restrepo, D.F.; García-Garro, P.A.; Castellote-Caballero, Y.; Achalandabaso-Ochoa, A.; Hita-Contreras, F. Enhancing Cognition in Older Adults with Mild Cognitive Impairment through High-Intensity Functional Training: A Single-Blind Randomized Controlled Trial. *J. Clin. Med.* **2023**, *12*, 4049. https://doi.org/10.3390/jcm12124049

Academic Editors: Yoshiaki Minakata and Kazuhisa Asai

Received: 14 May 2023
Revised: 10 June 2023
Accepted: 13 June 2023
Published: 14 June 2023

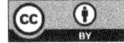

Copyright: © 2023 by the authors. Licensee MDPI, Basel, Switzerland. This article is an open access article distributed under the terms and conditions of the Creative Commons Attribution (CC BY) license (https://creativecommons.org/licenses/by/4.0/).

1. Introduction

Cognition, defined as the ability to learn, remember, solve problems and appropriately use previously stored information, is one of the most important factors in healthy aging [1].

Multiple complex structures are strongly affected by aging, generating neuroanatomical and neurophysiological changes that impact cognition [2]. One of the pathologies that are associated with cognition as a result of aging is mild cognitive impairment (MCI).

MCI is considered the transition point between the cognition problems expected during aging and dementia [3]. Although it is a relatively common disease, that affects between six and fifty million people worldwide with a prevalence that tends to double every five years [4], no pharmacological treatment exists yet that can prevent or cure it [5]. Considering that the decline in cognition has been multiple times negatively associated with the practice of physical activity [6,7] and that the prevalence of sedentary lifestyles along with life expectancy is increasing [8,9], it is logical to think that this disease will become a public health problem in the medium term.

Hence, many researchers have focused their attention on this pathology, seeking cost-effective treatments that can help to reduce the economic burden on the health systems that this disease represents. Among the possible interventions, physical exercise is highlighted for its effects on blood flow [10], oxidative stress [11] and brain volume [12], which could mitigate the impact of aging and thus delay the onset of diseases that lead to cognitive impairment.

Several authors have investigated the effects of physical activity on variables associated with cognition, such as verbal fluency, processing speed, and selective attention, and have observed favorable results in the older adult population [13,14]. In recent years, there has been an increasing recognition that these cognitive variables can serve as predictors of cognitive impairment, enabling early diagnosis and a more accurate prognosis [15]. Consequently, it is widely considered that exercise practice generates positive effects on cognition in older adults with MCI.

One training method that has gained particular attention is the high-intensity and short-duration training, known as High-Intensity Interval Training (HIIT) or its variant High-Intensity Functional Training (HIFT), which, unlike HIIT, focuses on the execution of multi-joint exercises with a functional approach that can be adapted to any level of physical condition [16]. HIFT programs have already been shown to be useful as a means of improving gait speed, strength, quality of life, muscle function and metabolic performance [17–19], among others in different populations, but their effects on cognition in older adults with MCI are still unclear [20]. Therefore, this study seeks to determine the effects of HIFT on different variables associated with cognition in Colombian older adults with MCI.

2. Materials and Methods

2.1. Study Design

This randomized controlled clinical trial (NCT04638322) was performed following the guidelines of the Consolidated Standards of Reporting Trials (CONSORT), with the approval of the Institutional Ethics Committee of the University of Jaén (SEP.20/4.TES) and in compliance with the Declaration of Helsinki. All participants signed an informed consent form.

2.2. Participants

The study participants were men and women over 65 years of age with MCI residing in five private institutions that offer care services for the elderly (nursing homes) in the city of Santiago de Cali, Colombia. Recruitment was carried out between January and March 2023 through direct visits in which the project was presented to each institution and the users and their families could decide whether to participate in the study. Each participant was screened with the MMSE to verify that he/she met the required cognitive level.

Participants were included if they met the following criteria: (i) being 65 years of age or older, (ii) voluntary acceptance of participation and signature of informed consent and (iii) having sufficient autonomy to perform physical activities and the ability to follow instructions. Exclusion criteria for this study were: (i) people performing some other exercise program, (ii) contraindicated for performing exercise or physical tests, (iii) medicated with beta-blockers, (iv) diagnosed with moderate or severe cognitive impairment, cancer, pulmonary hypertension, renal failure, heart failure, infected with Human Immunodeficiency Virus (HIV/AIDS), orphan diseases or with neurological disorders and (v) the population that does not accept participation or refuses the use of their data for the research.

2.3. Procedures

Randomization was carried out systematically using Epidat 4.2 software (Xunta de Galicia, Consellería de Sanidade-Servizo Galego de Saúde, Spain); additionally, to guarantee blinding, different work teams were organized: one for recruitment and admission of participants, another for the execution of the intervention, and another for pre- and post-measurements. Likewise, the analysis of the results was performed by an epidemiologist who was not involved in the previous process and who received the database in a coded form to keep the information confidential and avoid distinction between the control group and the experimental group.

The sample size was determined with a confidence level of 95% and a power of 90%, with an expected improvement of 10 points in the mean of each measurement in the intervention group (IG). The sample size was 120 people, divided into two balanced groups of 60 people each (60 for the control group and 60 for the intervention group). In addition, this value was adjusted to a probable loss rate of 20%, for which 145 persons were randomized.

2.4. Outcomes

Sociodemographic data, including sex, age, socioeconomic strata (according to Law 142 of 1994 that establishes the Regime of Domiciliary Public Services in Colombia), education level, occupation and tobacco and alcohol consumption, was collected through surveys. This data obtained through surveys were then cross-verified and confirmed with the participants' own registration forms, which were submitted upon their admission to the nursing home.

Cognition was assessed in participants using the following validated scales:

General cognition was assessed with the Montreal cognitive assessment/MoCA test, which evaluated executive and visuospatial function, memory, attention, language, abstraction, recall and orientation [21].

Attention and executive functions were assessed through the Trail Making Test part A and part B (TMTA and TMTB, respectively), which consists of visual and timed motor tasks where participants had to connect consecutively numbered circles (TMTA) or alternating circles of numbers and letters (TMTB) [22]. The shorter the time in which the person manages to connect all the circles, the better the level of attention and executive function is considered [23].

For verbal fluency, the Verbal Fluency Test (VFT) was applied; this test is widely used worldwide in neuropsychological evaluation. The instrument consists of asking the patient to name as many animals as possible for one minute, without using superordinate categories, such as fish, or subordinate categories [24].

Selective attention and concentration were assessed with the D2 test. Selective attention focuses on the subject's ability to quickly discriminate and select a specific visual stimulus (i.e., the letter "d" with two marks) among other randomly appearing distractor stimuli. This is a time-limited test of following instructions that considers the ability to discriminate stimuli. The output scores are divided into total hits (TH), percentage error (%E), total test effectiveness (TE), calculated from the difference between total words processed and errors, and the concentration index (CON), obtained from the difference between TH and commission errors (errors made by mistakenly marking a letter as correct when it should have been omitted). This test is a useful instrument in research, showing a high degree of validity and reliability [25].

Processing speed was assessed through the Digit Symbol Substitution Test (DSST), a paper-and-pencil cognitive test, presented on a single sheet of paper that requires a subject to match symbols to numbers according to a key located at the top of the page. The subject copies the symbol in spaces below a row of numbers. The number of correct symbols within the time allowed, usually 90 to 120 s, constitutes the score [26]. The maximum score is 60.

2.5. Intervention

Two groups were defined in this study.

The intervention group (IG) received a HIFT program for 12 weeks with 3 sessions per week, with a duration of 45 min per session. The sessions were led by a professional in sports science. The exercises to be performed were divided into three phases. Warm-up: 10 min of joint mobility, starting with neck flexion-extension, rotation and lateral flexion-inflection while looking at a fixed point. Trunk mobility exercises executing rotations were performed. For the upper limb, flexion, extension, abduction, and adduction, as well as internal and external rotation, grip exercises and pumping exercises were performed. For the lower limb, hip abduction and adduction from a standing position with upper limb support on the table, as well as hip and knee extension, plantar flexion and ankle dorsiflexion were performed.

The main part consisted of 25 min divided into 4 intervals of 4 min each, performed at an intensity of 80–85% of the maximum heart rate. The exercises included a simulation of a bicycle exercise from a seated position with alternating lower limb movement, wall push-up from a standing position, chair squat with upper limb stabilization support and throwing and catching balls against the wall while performing lateral and frontal lunges. Each exercise was performed for 20 to 30 s as intensely or as fast as possible without generating joint impact, followed by a rest period of 10 to 15 s before repeating the exercise.

The return to calm consisted of 10 min of muscle stretching, with an emphasis on the quadriceps, gluteus maximus and gluteus medius, biceps and triceps brachii and gastrocnemius muscles.

The intervention was standardized and conducted at the group level, with subgroups of 10 people to facilitate logistics and heart rate control using heart rate monitors. Each assistant was assigned a maximum of 2 participants for supervision during the training phase and rest phase, ensuring the necessary intensity was reached.

During the first two weeks, an exercise adaptation protocol was carried out. For this, in the main phase, aerobic training was performed with an initial intensity of 50% to 60% of the maximum heart rate. After the third week, the exercises were divided into four 4 min intervals at an intensity of 80–90% of the maximum heart rate followed by active rest intervals of 3 min at 40–60% of the maximum heart rate. From the fourth week onwards, the exercises continued with the same distribution, but the intensity increased to 85–95% of the maximum heart rate followed by active rest intervals of 3 min at 50–70% of the maximum heart rate.

On the other hand, the control group (CG) participated in the execution of manual activities, such as painting mandalas on paper and decorating picture frames. These activities were directed by occupational therapists and supported logistically by nursing assistants. The CG engaged in these activities for 12 weeks, with a frequency of 3 sessions per week and a duration of 45 min each. Additionally, they were provided with the PAHO physical activity recommendations guide, which had been prepared by professionals in sports science.

2.6. Statistical Analysis

The population was characterized according to its socio-demographic conditions, differentiated by groups (CG and IG). Qualitative variables were presented with frequency and percentage in each category. Given the normal distribution of the cognitive outcome variables (Kolmogorov–Smirnov test $p > 0.05$), the data were presented with the mean value and standard deviation (SD). To ensure equality between groups in the initial conditions, chi-square and Student's *t*-test statistical tests were applied.

Intra-group analysis was performed with a paired *t*-test to evaluate changes in each cognitive test before and after the intervention. The effect size was measured using Cohen's d, where a value of ≤ 0.2 indicates no effect, >0.2 and ≤ 0.5 indicates a small effect, >0.5 and ≤ 0.8 indicates a medium effect and >0.8 indicates a large effect [27].

For the analysis of the comparison between IG and CG at the end of the intervention, the ANOVA test and the mixed ANOVA analysis were performed, with the factor between groups being participation in or absence from the HIFT program. Each dependent variable was evaluated with possible group-by-time interactions to determine if significant differences exist between the groups over time. The within-group factor was time, and the effect size was evaluated using eta-squared (η^2).

Finally, all the dependent variables of cognition were integrated into a multiple regression model adjusted for the covariates sex, age, initial MMSE level and education level. For all statistical hypothesis tests, a significance level of 0.05 and a confidence level of 95% were established and analyzed using the Stata 14.0 statistical package (STATA Corporation, College Station, TX, USA).

3. Results

From a total of 224 elderly residents in the institutions who were eligible, 145 were randomized and allocated to the CG ($n = 73$) and the IG ($n = 72$). During the follow-up, 13 persons dropped out of the study (5 in the CG and 8 in the IG). Finally, 132 patients participated in the study; refer to Figure 1.

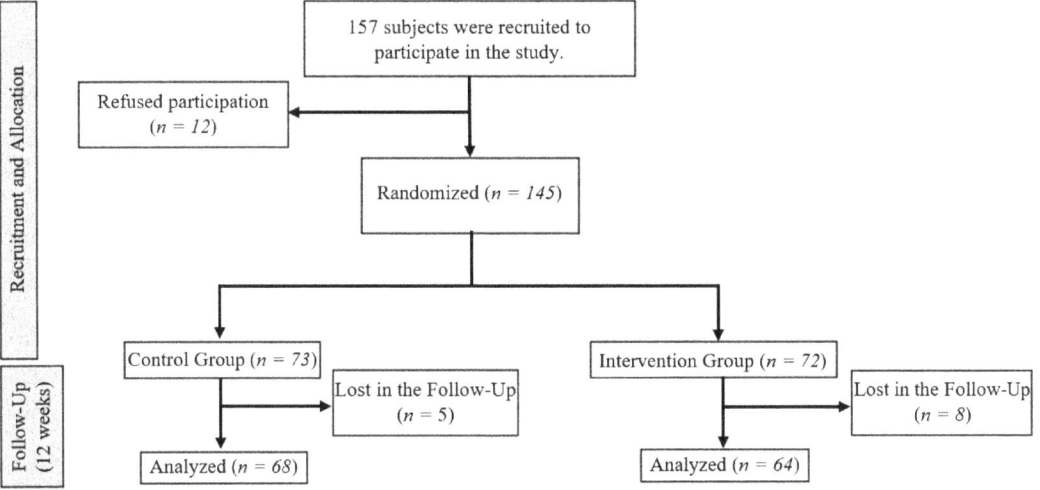

Figure 1. CONSORT flow diagram showing participant selection and allocation.

The sociodemographic characteristics (Table 1) show a participation rate of 59.8% females and 40.2% males in the population. They belonged to a middle socioeconomic stratum (36.4%), completed secondary education (53.0%) or professional education (28.8%), worked as housewives (41.7%) or were retired (31.8%); they did not use tobacco (95.5%) or consume alcohol (70.5%) and had an average age of 77.15 ± 7.67 years and an MMSE of 21.54 ± 1.42. None of the variables measured at baseline showed significant differences between the CG and IG ($p > 0.05$), which makes the intervention and post-intervention comparison feasible. Additionally, no adverse events were reported during the course of the investigation.

Table 1. Baseline characteristics of the participants (n = 132).

		Total (n = 132)	CG (n = 68)	IG (n = 64)	p Value
Age. Mean (SD)		77.2 (7.6)	77.19 (7.7)	77.11 (7.3)	0.951
MMSE. Mean (SD)		21.5 (1.37)	21.56 (1.25)	21.62 (1.59)	0.862
Sex. n (%)	Female	79 (59.8)	41 (60.3)	38 (59.4)	0.914
	Male	53 (40.2)	27 (39.7)	26 (40.6)	
Socioeconomic strata. n (%)	1	0 (0.0)	0 (0.0)	0 (0.0)	0.731
	2	0 (0.0)	0 (0.0)	0 (0.0)	
	3	45 (34.1)	26 (38.2)	19 (29.7)	
	4	48 (36.4)	23 (33.8)	25 (39.1)	
	5	22 (16.7)	10 (14.7)	12 (18.8)	
	6	17 (12.9)	9 (13.2)	8 (12.5)	
Education level. n (%)	Elementary school	21 (15.9)	12 (17.6)	9 (14.1)	0.862
	High school	70 (53.0)	35 (51.5)	35 (54.7)	
	College	38 (28.8)	20 (29.4)	18 (28.1)	
	Postgraduate	3 (2.3)	1 (1.5)	2 (3.1)	
Occupation. n (%)	Housewife	55 (41.7)	35 (51.5)	20 (31.3)	0.821
	Businessman	5 (3.8)	3 (4.4)	2 (3.1)	
	Self-employed	30 (22.7)	14 (20.6)	16 (25.0)	
	Employed	42 (31.8)	16 (23.5)	26 (40.6)	
Tobacco consumption. n (%)	No	126 (95.5)	63 (92.6)	63 (98.4)	0.115
	Yes	6 (4.5)	5 (7.4)	1 (1.6)	
Alcohol consumption. n (%)	No	93 (70.5)	46 (67.6)	47 (73.4)	0.466
	Yes	39 (29.5)	22 (32.4)	17 (26.6)	

SD: standard deviation; MMSE: mini-mental status examination; CG: control group; IG: intervention group; n: frequency.

3.1. General Cognition

Cognitive impairment measured on the MoCA scale initially showed a mean score of 21.53 ± 1.18 for the CG and 21.63 ± 1.53 for the IG (p = 0.687). Post-intervention, a mean difference of 0.902 was found (CG 21.68 ± 1.27 vs. IG 22.58 ± 1.41), which was statistically significant with a medium effect size ($p < 0.001$, Cohen's $d = -0.671$), highlighting higher scores in participants who received the HIFT program. The intra-group analysis paired t-test was -5.55 ($p < 0.001$, Cohen's $d = 0.694$). The group × time interaction analysis was also significant ($F = 5.87$ $p = 0.016$ $\eta^2 = 0.021$), which corroborates the effects of the HIFT intervention and its interaction with the measurement time (see Table 2).

Table 2. Effects of the HIFT program over the general cognition, psychomotor attention, attention and executive functions, verbal fluency and processing speed.

Test Mean (SD)	Pre			Post			Group			Time			Group × Time		
	CG	IG	p Value	CG	IG	p Value	F	p Value	η^2	F	p Value	η^2	F	p Value	η^2
MoCA TEST.	21.53 (1.18)	21.63 (1.53)	0.687	21.68 (1.27)	22.58 (1.41)	<0.001 **	8.98	0.003 *	0.031	10.93	0.001 *	0.038	5.87	0.016 *	0.021
TMTA	95.44 (10.47)	97.25 (12.71)	0.373	93.99 (10.37)	85.86 (10.72)	<0.001 **	5.35	0.021 *	0.018	22.13	<0.001 **	0.074	13.24	<0.001 **	0.044
TMTB	204.25 (38.60)	199.33 (29.09)	0.412	199.49 (41.91)	186.83 (24.12)	0.037 *	3.067	0.039 *	0.016	4155	0.043	0.015	0.834	0.362	0.003
VFT	20.19 (3.08)	19.92 (3.18)	0.622	22.2 (3.08)	25.8 (2.43)	<0.001 **	20.5	<0.001 **	0.048	115.6	<0.001 **	0.273	27.8	<0.001 **	0.065
D2	48.90 (9.88)	48.13 (10.45)	0.663	53.97 (14.29)	51.64 (12.12)	0.316	1.135	0.288	0.004	8.699	0.003 *	0.032	0.286	0.593	0.001
D2-TA	130.71 (17.78)	128.53 (16.02)	0.463	111.99 (19.34)	210.58 (41.56)	<0.001 **	20.8	<0.001 **	0.275	100	<0.001 **	0.118	254	<0.001 **	0.300

Table 2. Cont.

Test Mean (SD)	Pre			Post			Group			Time			Group × Time		
	CG	IG	p Value	CG	IG	p Value	F	p Value	η²	F	p Value	η²	F	p Value	η²
D2-%E	6.69 (2.30)	6.80 (1.92)	0.767	9.05 (3.38)	5.37 (2.55)	<0.001 **	31.05	<0.001 **	0.095	02.07	0.151	0.006	34.98	<0.001 **	0.107
D2-TOT	338.38 (51.86)	335.23 (51.74)	0.728	347.47 (67.37)	354.03 (57.74)	0.55	0.058	0.810	0.000	3.861	0.050	0.015	0.468	0.494	0.002
D2-CON	122.29 (18.32)	120.28 (15.93)	0.503	101.40 (20.53)	204.33 (43.39)	<0.001 **	235.5	<0.001 **	0.280	92.2	<0.001 **	0.109	254.7	<0.001 **	0.302
DSST	48.03 (7.63)	45.50 (8.61)	0.076	48.22 (7.56)	44.77 (9.69)	0.24	8.3808	0.004 *	0.031	0.069	0.793	0.000	0.201	0.655	0.001

MoCA: Montreal cognitive assessment; TMTA: Trail Making Test A; TMTB: Trail Making Test B; VFT: Verbal Fluency Test; %E: percentage of error; CON: concentration index; CG: control group; IG: intervention group; DSST: Digit Symbol Substitution Test. *: p value < 0.05; **: p values < 0.001.

3.2. Attention

The attention evaluated at the beginning of the research with the TMTA test, obtained time records of 95.44 ± 10.47 and 97.25 ± 12.71 s for the CG and IG, respectively. After the intervention, the measurements showed a decrease in the time taken to execute the test in the IG (85.86 ± 10.72), which demonstrates a significant improvement compared to the initial conditions ($p < 0.001$, mean difference = -0.953 Cohen's $d = 0.694$). When post-intervention comparison was made between groups, a difference of 8.12 s was observed, which proves that the intervention with HIFT favors attention and speed with a medium effect ($p < 0.001$, Cohen's $d = 0.771$). The ANCOVA analysis corroborated the group differences as a function of time ($F = 13.24$, $p < 0.001$, $\eta^2 = 0.044$)

3.3. Executive Functions

The executive functions assessed through the TMTB at baseline showed time records of 204.25 ± 38.60 for CG and 199.33 ± 29.09 for IG ($p = 0.412$). Once the intervention ended, the means of both groups decreased (CG = 199.49 ± 41.91 and IG = 186.83 ± 24.12) evidencing significant changes within each group, but with a small effect size in CG ($p = 0.027$, mean difference = 5.05, Cohen's $d = 0.274$) and large effect size in IG ($p < 0.001$, mean difference = 12.5, Cohen's $d = 0.880$). Consequently, the group × time analysis of covariance was not significant ($F = 0.834$ $p = 0.36$ $\eta^2 = 0.003$). The intergroup comparison of the final measurements showed that despite the fact that both showed improvement over time, the intervention with HIFT had a better outcome, but the effect size of this difference was small (mean difference between groups = 12.65, $p = 0.037$, Cohen's $d = 0.367$).

3.4. Verbal Fluency

The verbal fluency assessment through the VFT at baseline showed similar scores (CG = 20.19 ± 3.08 and IG = 19.92 ± 3.18; $p = 0.622$); after 12 weeks of intervention, significant differences were observed between the groups, evidencing the influence of HIFT in the increase of word registration in one minute and a large effect size (CG 22.2 ± 3.08; IG = 25.8 ± 2.43, mean diff = 3.574, $p < 0.001$, Cohen's $d = 1.284$). The pre- and post-comparison showed that the IG achieved a significant improvement in verbal fluency and its effect size is large ($p < 0.001$, mean difference = -5.844, Cohen's $d = -2.366$).

Considering the mixed variance group × time, it was possible to establish that significant differences exist between the groups as a function of time, showing changes in the IG that favor processing speed ($F = 27.8$, $p < 0.001$, $\eta^2 = 0.065$).

3.5. Selective Attention and Concentration

Post-intervention inter-group analysis of the D2 test percentile score (CG = 53.97 ± 14.2 and IG = 51.64 ± 12.1) showed neither significant differences (mean difference = 2.330, $p = 0.316$, Cohen's $d = 0.174$) nor intra-group analysis of the IG (mean difference = -3.516, $p = 0.095$, Cohen's $d = -0.212$). However, when analyzing the individual components of the D2, an increase in the TH with a large effect size (mean difference = −82.093, Cohen's d = −2.601), a decrease in the %E (mean difference = −8.73, $p < 0.001$) with large effect size (Cohen's d = 1.30) and an improvement in the CON (mean difference = −84.09, $p < 0.001$, Cohen's d = 2.53) can be observed in the intra-group comparison of the IG. Inter-group analyses for these variables also prove post-intervention differences in favor of the HIFT program ($p < 0.001$).

In the mixed variance analysis, no group × time interaction was observed (F = 0.286, p = 0.593, η^2 = 0.001), which indicates that neither the changes in time nor the group were significantly related for the d2 percentile, the total number of responses (F = 0.112, p = 0.738, η^2 = 0.000) or the total effectiveness of the test (F = 0.468, p = 0.494, η^2 = 0.002), although it did show an interaction for the TH (F = 254, $p < 0.001$, η^2 = 0.300), the %E (F = 34.98, $p < 0.001$, η^2 = 0.107) and the CON (F = 254.7, $p < 0.001$, η^2 = 0.302).

3.6. Processing Speed

Processing speed through DSST score (CG = 48.22 ± 7.56 and IG = 44.77 ± 9.69) did not show significant changes between groups after the intervention (mean difference between groups = 3.455, p = 0.24, Cohen's d = 0.399). Considering the mixed variance group × time, it could be determined that there were neither significant differences between groups as a function of time (F = 0.069, p = 0.793, η^2 = 0.000) nor significant interaction found (F = 0.201, $p < 0.655$, η^2 = 0.001).

The multivariate statistical analysis (MANCOVA) integrated all the cognitive variables (Moca, TMTA TMTB, d2, VFT and DSST) and found an interaction with the education level (p = 0.026) that favored those with higher levels of education. Adjustment for all sociodemographic variables was performed, which allowed establishing that the effects of the intervention evidenced in all cognitive variables are maintained independently of sex, age and MMSE level (F = 62.922, $p < 0.001$, Wilks' λ = 0.133) (Table 3).

Table 3. MANCOVA for MoCA, TMTA TMTB, d2, VFT and DSST for evaluation of interaction with MMSE, group assigned, education level, sex and age.

Model	Wilks' λ	F	p Value
GROUP	0.133	62.922	<0.001 **
EDUCATION LEVEL	0.670	1.379	0.087
SEX	0.938	0.631	0.796
GROUP × EDUCATION LEVEL	0.635	1.580	0.026 *
GROUP × SEX	0.932	0.710	0.730
EDUCATION LEVEL × SEX	0.906	0.493	0.976
GROUP × EDUCATION LEVEL × SEX	0.835	0.912	0.579
AGE	0.746	3.285	<0.001 **
MMSE	0.698	4.174	<0.001 **

MMSE: mini-mental status examination. *: p value < 0.05; **: p values < 0.001.

4. Discussion

The objective of this study was to determine the effect of a HIFT program on cognitive functions in a Colombian older adult population with MCI. Among the main findings, it was observed that HIFT is an effective strategy to improve general cognition, psychomotor speed and attention, executive functions and verbal fluency, although no significant differences were observed in concentration or information processing speed. Together, these findings corroborate the importance of physical exercise for the brain health of older adults. Considering that cognitive impairment and dementia have become a major burden for health systems, families and the community, in addition to the large financial costs it entails [28,29], this study is of great value, since it proposes new methods of early treatment of dementia to prevent the loss and even improve cognitive performance and quality of life of older adults.

The regular practice of a physical activity is being recognized as a highly protective factor of the cognitive functions [30] and for its neuroprotective effects on brain regions that are vulnerable to neurodegeneration, including the hippocampus and temporal and frontal regions [31–33]. Our findings revealed that a 12-week HIFT program improved general cognition in older adults with MCI; similarly, a study conducted on people with dementia in Nigeria [34] showed that a circuit training program is effective in improving, developing and training cognition [35]. Likewise, a randomized trial showed that a high-intensity strength training program, performed for four months significantly improved global cognitive function and maintained the benefits for eighteen months [35].

In relation to the processing speed evaluated with the DSST, no significant improvements were obtained. Consistent with these results, Zhu et al. [36] found that there was no correlation between the physical activity program and processing speed. A systematic review conducted on 809 people receiving interventions based on rhythmic physical activity concluded that the longer the intervention (>13 weeks) the better the effects on cognition [37]. This could explain the lack of significant differences in processing speed since the duration of the study was 12 weeks. It should be highlighted that, although there is evidence of the benefits of HIFT on cognition, due to the heterogeneity of the intervention protocols, it is still necessary to generate more research to determine the dose-response that guarantees the effectiveness of the interventions in relation to all the components of cognition [20].

In this research, attention and executive functions were evaluated through the TMTA and TMTB, respectively. The results showed significant improvements for both tests; however, selective attention and concentration evaluated with the D2 did not show significant differences. This dissimilarity could be explained by the fact that in the D2, attention is not considered as a single aptitude; for this reason, components such as processing speed, precision, stability, fatigue and the effectiveness of attentional inhibition are considered [25]. For the executive functions evaluated with the TMTB, significant changes were found for both CG and IG, with a small effect size for the CG (Cohen's d = 0.274) and a large effect size for the IG (Cohen's d = 0.880). This could be explained since therapies based on visual arts, such as the one proposed in this study in the control group, have been shown to be effective in improving cognitive functions [38,39]. Similarly, with the practice of physical exercise a stronger connectivity can be achieved between the amygdala and the medial temporal gyrus, inferior frontal gyrus, postcentral gyrus and hippocampus, regions that are related to memory and executive functions [40,41]. From these findings, it can be suggested that although it is common to prescribe activities involved with the arts and physical exercise in people with dementia [42], therapies that include physical exercise may be more effective.

Verbal fluency was another variable that showed significant improvements, which is consistent with a study conducted with postmenopausal women where improvements in verbal fluency were found after 12 weeks of Pilates training [43]. Similarly, a systematic review with meta-analysis suggests that physical exercise can produce improvements in verbal fluency in older adults with MCI [44]. It is possible that verbal fluency may be responsive to improvements from physical exercise interventions, especially aerobic exercise, due to the positive selective impact of this type of intervention on the frontal and prefrontal regions of the brain.

Likewise, high-intensity physical exercise has been shown to be more beneficial for brain health than moderate-intensity exercise because, although the physical exercise of different intensities has improvements in different aspects related to brain health, it is vigorous intensity exercise that has the greatest effects on acute levels of circulating brain-derived neurotrophic factor and corticospinal excitability [45,46]. Furthermore, it improves neural plasticity of the hippocampus [47,48], facilitates inhibitory control and its underlying neuro-electrical activation [49], improves brain activation during memory retrieval [50], decreases oxidative stress and anxiety levels and increases antioxidants capacity as a protective system against neuronal damage [51]. In addition, a high-intensity interval training session has a three times shorter duration than a continuous training session of low or moderate intensity [52], which implies a lower time cost while maximizing the beneficial effects at cardiovascular, metabolic and systemic levels [53].

Finally, this study had some limitations. First, the effects of HIFT were evaluated only in the short term, and the intervention time was short. Second, it was conducted only with adults living in the city of Santiago de Cali, Colombia; for this reason, the findings cannot be generalized to other populations. Third, it is important to develop more research that evaluates the effects of HIFT on cognition in older adults with MCI in the long term. And fourth, the lack of consideration for the co-occurrence of other medical conditions and the pharmacological treatments of the patients, apart from those mentioned in the exclusion criteria, could have potentially influenced the results. Among the strengths of this study, we can find its low attrition rate, in addition to its large sample size and its randomized, single-blinded, controlled trial design.

5. Conclusions

The present study, developed in Colombian older adults with MCI, demonstrates that a 12-week HIFT program with a frequency of 3 times per week has beneficial effects on general cognition, attention, executive functions and verbal fluency.

Considering that the population of older adults continues to grow and that the prevalence of dementia is increasing, it is important to generate strategies such as the one presented in this study. Similarly, further research on the effects of HIFT is needed to determine the most appropriate dose-response to improve cognition and its different components. In light of these considerations, it is imperative that future research endeavors concentrate on providing comprehensive descriptions of training variables, including volume, time and frequency. Moreover, conducting comparative studies between various training protocols will enable a thorough analysis of the aforementioned dose-response relationships.

Author Contributions: Conceptualization, Y.R.-C., Y.C.-C. and D.F.A.-R.; methodology, A.A.-A., A.A.-O. and P.A.G.-G.; formal analysis, Y.R.-C. and C.R.-L.; writing—original draft preparation, Y.C.-C., F.H.-C. and D.F.A.-R.; writing—review and editing, A.A.-O. and P.A.G.-G.; supervision, A.A.-A., F.H.-C. and C.R.-L. All authors have read and agreed to the published version of the manuscript.

Funding: This research received no external funding.

Institutional Review Board Statement: The study was conducted in accordance with the Declaration of Helsinki and approved by the Ethics Committee of the University of Jaén (14 October 2020).

Informed Consent Statement: Informed consent was obtained from all subjects involved in the study.

Data Availability Statement: The data presented in this study are available on request from the corresponding author. The data are not publicly available because, due to the sensitive nature of the questions asked in this study, participants were assured raw data would remain confidential and would not be shared.

Conflicts of Interest: The authors declare no conflict of interest.

References

1. Morley, J.E.; Morris, J.C.; Berg-Weger, M.; Borson, S.; Carpenter, B.D.; del Campo, N.; Dubois, B.; Fargo, K.; Fitten, L.J.; Flaherty, J.H.; et al. Brain Health: The Importance of Recognizing Cognitive Impairment: An IAGG Consensus Conference. *J. Am. Med. Dir. Assoc.* **2015**, *16*, 731–739. [CrossRef] [PubMed]
2. Jäncke, L.; Martin, M.; Röcke, C.; Mérillat, S. Editorial: Longitudinal aging research: Cognition, behavior and neuroscience. *Front. Hum. Neurosci.* **2022**, *16*, 1002560. [CrossRef] [PubMed]
3. Anderson, N.D. State of the science on mild cognitive impairment (MCI). *CNS Spectr.* **2019**, *24*, 78–87. [CrossRef] [PubMed]
4. Pérez Palmer, N.; Trejo Ortega, B.; Joshi, P. Cognitive Impairment in Older Adults: Epidemiology, Diagnosis, and Treatment. *Psychiatr. Clin. N. Am.* **2022**, *45*, 639–661. [CrossRef] [PubMed]
5. Sanford, A.M. Mild Cognitive Impairment. *Clin. Geriatr. Med.* **2017**, *33*, 325–337. [CrossRef]
6. Middleton, L.E.; Barnes, D.E.; Lui, L.Y.; Yaffe, K. Physical activity over the life course and its association with cognitive performance and impairment in old age. *J. Am. Geriatr. Soc.* **2010**, *58*, 1322–1326. [CrossRef]
7. Scarmeas, N.; Luchsinger, J.A.; Schupf, N.; Brickman, A.M.; Cosentino, S.; Tang, M.X.; Stern, Y. Physical activity, diet, and risk of Alzheimer disease. *JAMA* **2009**, *302*, 627–637. [CrossRef]
8. Rodulfo, J.I.A. Sedentary lifestyle a disease from XXI century. *Clin. Investig. Arterioscler. Publ. Off. Soc. Esp. Arterioscler.* **2019**, *31*, 233–240. [CrossRef]

9. GBD US Health Disparities Collaborators. Life expectancy by county, race, and ethnicity in the USA, 2000–2019: A systematic analysis of health disparities. *Lancet* **2022**, *400*, 25–38. [CrossRef]
10. De la Rosa, A.; Olaso-Gonzalez, G.; Arc-Chagnaud, C.; Millan, F.; Salvador-Pascual, A.; García-Lucerga, C.; Blasco-Lafarga, C.; Garcia-Dominguez, E.; Carretero, A.; Correas, A.G.; et al. Physical exercise in the prevention and treatment of Alzheimer's disease. *J. Sport Health Sci.* **2020**, *9*, 394–404. [CrossRef]
11. Gomes, M.J.; Martinez, P.F.; Pagan, L.U.; Damatto, R.L.; Cezar, M.D.M.; Lima, A.R.R.; Okoshi, K.; Okoshi, M.P. Skeletal muscle aging: Influence of oxidative stress and physical exercise. *Oncotarget* **2017**, *8*, 20428–20440. [CrossRef] [PubMed]
12. López, M.D.; Zamarrón, M.D.; Fernández-Ballesteros, R. Relationship between exercising and physical and cognitive function indicators. Comparison of results with age. *Rev. Esp. Geriatr. Gerontol.* **2011**, *46*, 15–20. [CrossRef]
13. Welford, P.; Östh, J.; Hoy, S.; Rossell, S.L.; Pascoe, M.; Diwan, V.; Hallgren, M. Effects of Yoga and Aerobic Exercise on Verbal Fluency in Physically Inactive Older Adults: Randomized Controlled Trial (FitForAge). *Clin. Interv. Aging* **2023**, *18*, 533–545. [CrossRef] [PubMed]
14. Liu-Ambrose, T.; Davis, J.C.; Falck, R.S.; Best, J.R.; Dao, E.; Vesely, K.; Ghag, C.; Rosano, C.; Hsu, C.L.; Dian, L.; et al. Exercise, Processing Speed, and Subsequent Falls: A Secondary Analysis of a 12-Month Randomized Controlled Trial. *J. Gerontol. Ser. A Biol. Sci. Med. Sci.* **2021**, *76*, 675–682. [CrossRef]
15. Ayers, M.R.; Bushnell, J.; Gao, S.; Unverzagt, F.; Gaizo, J.D.; Wadley, V.G.; Kennedy, R.; Clark, D.G. Verbal fluency response times predict incident cognitive impairment. *Alzheimer's Dement.* **2022**, *14*, e12277. [CrossRef] [PubMed]
16. Feito, Y.; Heinrich, K.M.; Butcher, S.J.; Poston, W.S.C. High-Intensity Functional Training (HIFT): Definition and Research Implications for Improved Fitness. *Sports* **2018**, *6*, 76. [CrossRef] [PubMed]
17. Buckley, S.; Knapp, K.; Lackie, A.; Lewry, C.; Horvey, K.; Benko, C.; Trinh, J.; Butcher, S. Multimodal high-intensity interval training increases muscle function and metabolic performance in females. *Appl. Physiol. Nutr. Metab. Physiol. Appl. Nutr. Metab.* **2015**, *40*, 1157–1162. [CrossRef] [PubMed]
18. Jiménez-García, J.D.; Martínez-Amat, A.; De la Torre-Cruz, M.J.; Fábrega-Cuadros, R.; Cruz-Díaz, D.; Aibar-Almazán, A.; Achalandabaso-Ochoa, A.; Hita-Contreras, F. Suspension Training HIIT Improves Gait Speed, Strength and Quality of Life in Older Adults. *Int. J. Sport. Med.* **2019**, *40*, 116–124. [CrossRef]
19. Peixoto, R.P.; Trombert, V.; Poncet, A.; Kizlik, J.; Gold, G.; Ehret, G.; Trombetti, A.; Reny, J.L. Feasibility and safety of high-intensity interval training for the rehabilitation of geriatric inpatients (HIITERGY) a pilot randomized study. *BMC Geriatr.* **2020**, *20*, 197. [CrossRef]
20. Rivas-Campo, Y.; García-Garro, P.A.; Aibar-Almazán, A.; Martínez-Amat, A.; Vega-Ávila, G.C.; Afanador-Restrepo, D.F.; León-Morillas, F.; Hita-Contreras, F. The Effects of High-Intensity Functional Training on Cognition in Older Adults with Cognitive Impairment: A Systematic Review. *Healthcare* **2022**, *10*, 670. [CrossRef]
21. Pedraza, O.L.; Salazar, A.M.; Sierra, F.A.; Soler, D.; Castro, J.; Castillo, P.C.; Hernandez, M.A.; Piñeros, C. Confiabilidad, validez de criterio y discriminante del Montreal Cognitive Assessment (MoCA) test, en un grupo de Adultos de Bogotá. *Acta Médica Colomb.* **2017**, *41*, 221–228. [CrossRef]
22. Reitan, R.M. Validity of the Trail Making Test as an Indicator of Organic Brain Damage. *Percept. Mot. Ski.* **1958**, *8*, 271–276. [CrossRef]
23. Ryan, J.; Carrière, I.; Amieva, H.; Rouaud, O.; Berr, C.; Ritchie, K.; Scarabin, P.Y.; Ancelin, M.L. Prospective analysis of the association between estrogen receptor gene variants and the risk of cognitive decline in elderly women. *Eur. Neuropsychopharmacol. J. Eur. Coll. Neuropsychopharmacol.* **2013**, *23*, 1763–1768. [CrossRef]
24. Isaacs, B.; Kennie, A.T. The Set test as an aid to the detection of dementia in old people. *Br. J. Psychiatry J. Ment. Sci.* **1973**, *123*, 467–470. [CrossRef] [PubMed]
25. Brickenkamp, R.; Cubero, N.S. *D2: Test de Atención*; Tea: Madrid, Spain, 2002.
26. Jaeger, J. Digit Symbol Substitution Test: The Case for Sensitivity Over Specificity in Neuropsychological Testing. *J. Clin. Psychopharmacol.* **2018**, *38*, 513–519. [CrossRef] [PubMed]
27. Cohen, J. *Statistical Power Analysis for the Behavioral Sciences*, 2nd ed.; Baskı: Hillsdale, NJ, USA, 1988.
28. Sugano, K.; Yokogawa, M.; Yuki, S.; Dohmoto, C.; Yoshita, M.; Hamaguchi, T.; Yanase, D.; Iwasa, K.; Komai, K.; Yamada, M. Effect of cognitive and aerobic training intervention on older adults with mild or no cognitive impairment: A derivative study of the nakajima project. *Dement. Geriatr. Cogn. Disord. Extra* **2012**, *2*, 69–80. [CrossRef]
29. Mattap, S.M.; Mohan, D.; McGrattan, A.M.; Allotey, P.; Stephan, B.C.; Reidpath, D.D.; Siervo, M.; Robinson, L.; Chaiyakunapruk, N. The economic burden of dementia in low- and middle-income countries (LMICs): A systematic review. *BMJ Glob. Health* **2022**, *7*, e007409. [CrossRef]
30. Tari, A.R.; Norevik, C.S.; Scrimgeour, N.R.; Kobro-Flatmoen, A.; Storm-Mathisen, J.; Bergersen, L.H.; Wrann, C.D.; Selbæk, G.; Kivipelto, M.; Moreira, J.B.N.; et al. Are the neuroprotective effects of exercise training systemically mediated? *Prog. Cardiovasc. Dis.* **2019**, *62*, 94–101. [CrossRef]
31. Domingos, C.; Pêgo, J.M.; Santos, N.C. Effects of physical activity on brain function and structure in older adults: A systematic review. *Behav. Brain Res.* **2021**, *402*, 113061. [CrossRef]
32. Falck, R.S.; Hsu, C.L.; Best, J.R.; Li, L.C.; Egbert, A.R.; Liu-Ambrose, T. Not Just for Joints: The Associations of Moderate-to-Vigorous Physical Activity and Sedentary Behavior with Brain Cortical Thickness. *Med. Sci. Sport. Exerc.* **2020**, *52*, 2217–2223. [CrossRef]

33. Moreno, C.; Wykes, T.; Galderisi, S.; Nordentoft, M.; Crossley, N.; Jones, N.; Cannon, M.; Correll, C.U.; Byrne, L.; Carr, S.; et al. How mental health care should change as a consequence of the COVID-19 pandemic. *Lancet Psychiatry* **2020**, *7*, 813–824. [CrossRef]
34. Gbiri, C.A.O.; Amusa, B.F. Progressive task-oriented circuit training for cognition, physical functioning and societal participation in individuals with dementia. *Physiother. Res. Int. J. Res. Clin. Phys. Ther.* **2020**, *25*, e1866. [CrossRef]
35. Singh, M.A.F.; Gates, N.; Saigal, N.; Wilson, G.C.; Meiklejohn, J.; Brodaty, H.; Wen, W.; Singh, N.; Baune, B.T.; Suo, C.; et al. The Study of Mental and Resistance Training (SMART) study—Resistance training and/or cognitive training in mild cognitive impairment: A randomized, double-blind, double-sham controlled trial. *J. Am. Med. Dir. Assoc.* **2014**, *15*, 873–880. [CrossRef]
36. Zhu, Y.; Gao, Y.; Guo, C.; Qi, M.; Xiao, M.; Wu, H.; Ma, J.; Zhong, Q.; Ding, H.; Zhou, Q.; et al. Effect of 3-Month Aerobic Dance on Hippocampal Volume and Cognition in Elderly People With Amnestic Mild Cognitive Impairment: A Randomized Controlled Trial. *Front. Aging Neurosci.* **2022**, *14*, 771413. [CrossRef]
37. Vega-Ávila, G.C.; Afanador-Restrepo, D.F.; Rivas-Campo, Y.; García-Garro, P.A.; Hita-Contreras, F.; Carcelén-Fraile, M.D.C.; Castellote-Caballero, Y.; Aibar-Almazán, A. Rhythmic Physical Activity and Global Cognition in Older Adults with and without Mild Cognitive Impairment: A Systematic Review. *Int. J. Environ. Res. Public Health* **2022**, *19*, 12230. [CrossRef]
38. Masika, G.M.; Yu, D.S.F.; Li, P.W.C. Visual art therapy as a treatment option for cognitive decline among older adults. A systematic review and meta-analysis. *J. Adv. Nurs.* **2020**, *76*, 1892–1910. [CrossRef] [PubMed]
39. Broadhouse, K.M.; Singh, M.F.; Suo, C.; Gates, N.; Wen, W.; Brodaty, H.; Jain, N.; Wilson, G.C.; Meiklejohn, J.; Singh, N.; et al. Hippocampal plasticity underpins long-term cognitive gains from resistance exercise in MCI. *NeuroImage Clin.* **2020**, *25*, 102182. [CrossRef] [PubMed]
40. Varma, V.R.; Tang, X.; Carlson, M.C. Hippocampal sub-regional shape and physical activity in older adults. *Hippocampus* **2016**, *26*, 1051–1060. [CrossRef] [PubMed]
41. Barha, C.K.; Best, J.R.; Rosano, C.; Yaffe, K.; Catov, J.M.; Liu-Ambrose, T. Sex-Specific Relationship Between Long-Term Maintenance of Physical Activity and Cognition in the Health ABC Study: Potential Role of Hippocampal and Dorsolateral Prefrontal Cortex Volume. *J. Gerontol. Ser. A Biol. Sci. Med. Sci.* **2020**, *75*, 764–770. [CrossRef] [PubMed]
42. Regier, N.G.; Hodgson, N.A.; Gitlin, L.N. Characteristics of Activities for Persons With Dementia at the Mild, Moderate, and Severe Stages. *Gerontologist* **2017**, *57*, 987–997. [CrossRef] [PubMed]
43. García-Garro, P.A.; Hita-Contreras, F.; Martínez-Amat, A.; Achalandabaso-Ochoa, A.; Jiménez-García, J.D.; Cruz-Díaz, D.; Aibar-Almazán, A. Effectiveness of A Pilates Training Program on Cognitive and Functional Abilities in Postmenopausal Women. *Int. J. Environ. Res. Public Health* **2020**, *17*, 3580. [CrossRef] [PubMed]
44. Biazus-Sehn, L.F.; Schuch, F.B.; Firth, J.; Stigger, F.S. Effects of physical exercise on cognitive function of older adults with mild cognitive impairment: A systematic review and meta-analysis. *Arch. Gerontol. Geriatr.* **2020**, *89*, 104048. [CrossRef] [PubMed]
45. Boyne, P.; Meyrose, C.; Westover, J.; Whitesel, D.; Hatter, K.; Reisman, D.S.; Cunningham, D.; Carl, D.; Jansen, C.; Khoury, J.C.; et al. Exercise intensity affects acute neurotrophic and neurophysiological responses poststroke. *J. Appl. Physiol.* **2019**, *126*, 431–443. [CrossRef] [PubMed]
46. O'Callaghan, A.; Harvey, M.; Houghton, D.; Gray, W.K.; Weston, K.L.; Oates, L.L.; Romano, B.; Walker, R.W. Comparing the influence of exercise intensity on brain-derived neurotrophic factor serum levels in people with Parkinson's disease: A pilot study. *Aging Clin. Exp. Res.* **2020**, *32*, 1731–1738. [CrossRef]
47. Dos Santos, J.R.; Bortolanza, M.; Ferrari, G.D.; Lanfredi, G.P.; do Nascimento, G.C.; Azzolini, A.; Del Bel, E.; de Campos, A.C.; Faça, V.M.; Vulczak, A.; et al. One-Week High-Intensity Interval Training Increases Hippocampal Plasticity and Mitochondrial Content without Changes in Redox State. *Antioxidants* **2020**, *9*, 445. [CrossRef]
48. De Lima, N.S.; De Sousa, R.A.L.; Amorim, F.T.; Gripp, F.; Diniz, E.M.C.O.; Henrique Pinto, S.; Peixoto, M.F.D.; Monteiro-Junior, R.S.; Bourbeau, K.; Cassilhas, R.C. Moderate-intensity continuous training and high-intensity interval training improve cognition, and BDNF levels of middle-aged overweight men. *Metab. Brain Dis.* **2022**, *37*, 463–471. [CrossRef]
49. Kao, S.C.; Westfall, D.R.; Soneson, J.; Gurd, B.; Hillman, C.H. Comparison of the acute effects of high-intensity interval training and continuous aerobic walking on inhibitory control. *Psychophysiology* **2017**, *54*, 1335–1345. [CrossRef]
50. Kao, S.C.; Wang, C.H.; Kamijo, K.; Khan, N.; Hillman, C. Acute effects of highly intense interval and moderate continuous exercise on the modulation of neural oscillation during working memory. *Int. J. Psychophysiol. Off. J. Int. Organ. Psychophysiol.* **2021**, *160*, 10–17. [CrossRef]
51. Koyuncuoğlu, T.; Sevim, H.; Çetrez, N.; Meral, Z.; Gönenç, B.; Dertsiz, E.K.; Akakın, D.; Yüksel, M.; Çakır, Ö.K. High intensity interval training protects from Post Traumatic Stress Disorder induced cognitive impairment. *Behav. Brain Res.* **2021**, *397*, 112923. [CrossRef]
52. Nicolò, A.; Girardi, M. The physiology of interval training: A new target to HIIT. *J. Physiol.* **2016**, *594*, 7169–7170. [CrossRef]
53. Calverley, T.A.; Ogoh, S.; Marley, C.J.; Steggall, M.; Marchi, N.; Brassard, P.; Lucas, S.J.E.; Cotter, J.D.; Roig, M.; Ainslie, P.N.; et al. HIITing the brain with exercise: Mechanisms, consequences and practical recommendations. *J. Physiol.* **2020**, *598*, 2513–2530. [CrossRef] [PubMed]

Disclaimer/Publisher's Note: The statements, opinions and data contained in all publications are solely those of the individual author(s) and contributor(s) and not of MDPI and/or the editor(s). MDPI and/or the editor(s) disclaim responsibility for any injury to people or property resulting from any ideas, methods, instructions or products referred to in the content.

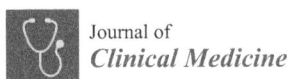

Article

Enhanced Physical Capacity and Gastrointestinal Symptom Improvement in Southern Italian IBS Patients following Three Months of Moderate Aerobic Exercise

Antonella Bianco [1,†], Francesco Russo [2,*,†], Isabella Franco [1], Giuseppe Riezzo [2], Rossella Donghia [3], Ritanna Curci [1], Caterina Bonfiglio [1], Laura Prospero [2], Benedetta D'Attoma [2], Antonia Ignazzi [2], Angelo Campanella [1] and Alberto Ruben Osella [1]

[1] Laboratory of Epidemiology and Statistics, National Institute of Gastroenterology IRCCS "Saverio de Bellis", 70013 Castellana Grotte, Italy; antonella.bianco@irccsdebellis.it (A.B.); isabella.franco@irccsdebellis.it (I.F.); ritanna.curci@irccsdebellis.it (R.C.); catia.bonfiglio@irccsdebellis.it (C.B.); angelo.campanella@irccsdebellis.it (A.C.); arosella@irccsdebellis.it (A.R.O.)

[2] Functional Gastrointestinal Disorders Research Group, National Institute of Gastroenterology IRCCS "Saverio de Bellis", 70013 Castellana Grotte, Italy; giuseppe.riezzo@irccsdebellis.it (G.R.); laura.prospero@irccsdebellis.it (L.P.); benedetta.dattoma@irccsdebellis.it (B.D.); antonia.ignazzi@irccsdebellis.it (A.I.)

[3] Data Science Unit, National Institute of Gastroenterology IRCCS "Saverio de Bellis", 70013 Castellana Grotte, Italy; rossella.donghia@irccsdebellis.it

* Correspondence: francesco.russo@irccsdebellis.it; Tel.: +39-080-4994-129; Fax: +39-080-4994-313

† These authors equally contributed to the work.

Abstract: Moderate-intensity aerobic exercise improves gastrointestinal (GI) health and alleviates irritable bowel syndrome (IBS) symptoms. This study explored its effects on physical capacity (PC) and IBS symptoms in 40 patients from Southern Italy (11 males, 29 females; 52.10 ± 7.72 years). The exercise program involved moderate-intensity aerobic exercise (60/75% of HRmax) for at least 180 min per week. Before and after the intervention, participants completed the IBS-SSS questionnaire to assess IBS symptoms, reported their physical activity levels, and underwent field tests to evaluate PC. PC was quantified as the Global Physical Capacity Score (GPCS). A total of 38 subjects (21 males, 17 females; 53.71 ± 7.27 years) without lower GI symptoms served as a No IBS group. No significant differences were found between IBS patients and No IBS subjects, except for the symptom score, as expected. After the exercise, all participants experienced significant improvements in both IBS symptoms and PC. Higher PC levels correlated with greater benefits in IBS symptomatology, especially with GPCS reaching above-average values. Engaging in moderate-intensity aerobic exercise for at least 180 min per week positively impacts IBS symptoms and PC. Monitoring GPCS in IBS patients provides insights into the connection between physical activity and symptom severity, aiding healthcare professionals in tailoring effective treatment plans.

Keywords: aerobic exercise; irritable bowel syndrome; Global Physical Capacity Score; physical capacity

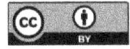

1. Introduction

Irritable bowel syndrome (IBS) is a prevalent functional gastrointestinal (GI) disorder, affecting approximately 9–22% of the European adult population [1,2]. This syndrome is characterized by abdominal pain or discomfort linked to altered bowel habits without an identifiable organic cause [3]. In addition to pharmacological treatments, there has been growing interest in alternative approaches to manage this condition better. Some of the most effective alternative treatments for IBS include acupuncture, herbal remedies, and mind–body techniques [4]. Peppermint oil, ginger, and aloe have been widely used as herbal remedies for treating IBS [5]. Psyllium powder and L-Glutamine have also been considered alternative natural remedies that may help with IBS [6]. Acupuncture has proven effective for treating chronic pain, but the studies are mixed on whether this treatment works for IBS [7].

Food is often considered a triggering factor for IBS symptoms, and diet is crucial to preventing and managing this functional disorder. However, there is no one-size-fits-all diet for individuals with IBS. Nonetheless, several dietary changes can help alleviate symptoms. Avoiding caffeine, alcohol, fatty foods, and spicy foods can also be helpful for some IBS patients [8]. Several studies have shown that a low FODMAPs (fermentable oligo-, di-, monosaccharides, and polyols) diet leads to a clinical response in 50–80% of IBS patients, particularly improving bloating, flatulence, and diarrhea [9]. In this context, our research group recently published articles highlighting the benefits of a low FODMAP diet [10] and a diet based on products derived from a new cereal called tritordeum [11]. Both dietary approaches have significantly improved GI symptoms.

As widely documented in the literature, physical activity (PA) plays a key role in the prevention and treatment of various diseases [12–15], can improve general health, and reduce stress levels. In addition, it exerts numerous positive and protective effects on the GI tract [16,17], such as relieving constipation [18] and improving digestive processes by increasing the speed of stool movement. Furthermore, Villoria et al. [19] demonstrated that PA reduces symptoms such as abdominal bloating by increasing intestinal gas clearance. The same group [20] previously demonstrated that PA improved gas transit and abdominal distension in healthy subjects but not the perception of bloating. A long-term follow-up study [21] showed that a placebo effect alone cannot explain PA's effects. A pure placebo effect would have to be decreased during follow-up.

From this perspective, PA can be a valuable tool for managing IBS, as increased participation in moderate PA has been associated with improved IBS symptoms. Several studies on IBS recommend an average prescription of 30 to 60 min of moderate-intensity aerobic PA, 3 to 5 times per week, for a minimum of 12 weeks [17]. Walking is the most common form of exercise, often complementary to other physical exercises [22]. It is known that regular walking, independent of other types of physical exercise, can improve risk factors for cardiovascular diseases, including diastolic blood pressure and lipid profiles, and reduces the risk of general mortality [23–25] and type 2 diabetes [26], and brings additional benefits in that it improves self-esteem, alleviates symptoms of depression and anxiety, and improves mood [27,28]. The advantages of using walking as a therapeutic tool are numerous: it can be performed at different speeds (and thus intensities), easily monitored by heart rate monitors, in groups or alone, and without special equipment or clothing.

In this framework, the walking group is a potentially interesting PA intervention as the dynamics and social cohesion of walking groups can have supportive effects that encourage and sustain adherence and positive attitudes towards PA [29], companionship, and the shared experience of well-being [30].

Regular walking, as well as regular PA, has many health effects related to physical capacity (PC) and can be assessed using various field tests. Unlike PA, which is related to the movements that people perform, PC is a set of attributes that people have or can achieve. The components of PC related to health [31] are: (a) cardiorespiratory capacity, (b) muscular resistance endurance, (c) muscle strength, (d) body composition, and (e) flexibility.

PC has been identified as an indicator of general health [32] and could also be a possible predictor of the response to PA treatment in IBS patients.

Based on the published evidence, we hypothesized that a programmed and controlled PA intervention could lead to an overall benefit in patients with IBS. In this framework, the study aimed to estimate the effect of a standardized PA program on the intensity and frequency of GI symptoms and the PC of IBS patients in Southern Italy.

2. Materials and Methods

2.1. Participants

Subjects were recruited in the study by the Functional Gastrointestinal Disorders Research Group in collaboration with the Laboratory of Epidemiology and Statistics of the National Institute of Gastroenterology IRCCS "Saverio de Bellis" Castellana Grotte, Italy. The project started in May 2022 and is still ongoing. The trial was registered at www.clinicaltrial.gov (accessed on 08 July 2022) (registration number NCT05453084).

2.2. Study Design

This study included adults attending the Outpatient Clinic for Celiac Disease and Functional Disorders who met the Rome III-IV criteria for IBS or were referred by local General Practitioners. The inclusion criteria were: (1) age 18–65 years, (2) availability to participate in the walking group, (3) in possession of a medical certificate of non-competitive sports fitness; and the exclusion criteria comprised: (1) presence of serious cardiac, hepatic, neurological or psychiatric diseases, (2) gastrointestinal disorders other than IBS, (3) subjects who have previously followed a low FODMAPs, vegan or gluten-free diet, (4) patients using antidepressants (5) significant orthopedic or neuromuscular limitations, (6) absolute contraindications to exercise. Furthermore, subjects who missed more than 20% of their training sessions would have been excluded from the analysis.

The study was conducted following the Helsinki Declaration and approved by the local Ethics Committee (Prot. N. 167/CE De Bellis).

2.3. Data Collection

During enrollment, participants signed informed consent and completed a structured questionnaire collecting data about sociodemographic aspects, medical history, and lifestyle. PA information was collected using the validated International Physical Activity Questionnaire, Short Form (IPAQ-SF) [33]. Patients also completed the symptom questionnaires Gastrointestinal Symptom Rating Scale (GSRS) for screening patients with IBS. The IBS-Severity Scoring System—IBS-SSS was administered to evaluate the selected patients' symptom intensity and frequency scores. Trained staff collected fast blood samples for biochemical assessments, anthropometric measurements (weight, height, waist circumference), and bio-impedance analysis. All measurements were taken at the start of the project and after 90 days. The timeline of the study design is shown in Figure 1.

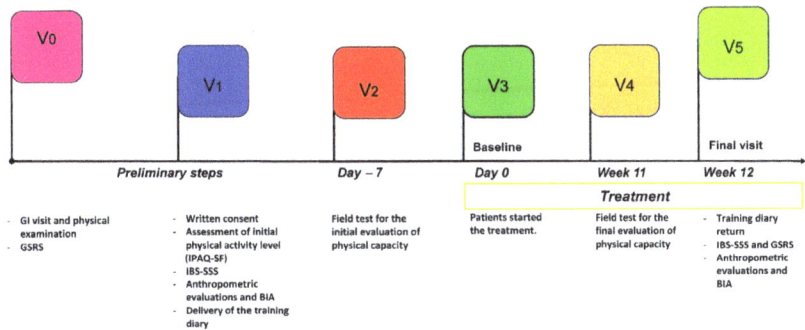

Figure 1. Study Design Timeline; GI: gastrointestinal; GSRS: Gastrointestinal Symptom Rating Scale; IBS-SSS: IBS-Severity Scoring System; BIA: bioelectrical impedance analysis.

2.4. Anthropometric and Bioelectrical Impedance Analysis (BIA) Parameters

The study assessed various anthropometric parameters to investigate the subjects' physical characteristics. The parameters included height, weight, body mass index (BMI), mid-upper arm, waist, and hip circumferences. Accurate measurements were obtained using a SECA 700 mechanical column scale and a SECA 220 altimeter (INTERMED S.r.l., Milan, Italy) for weight and height assessment, facilitating the subsequent calculation of BMI (kg/m^2).

To ensure uniformity, a stringent protocol was followed for individuals undergoing bioelectrical impedance analysis (BIA). All participants observed a minimum 4 h fasting period and refrained from alcohol consumption and strenuous exercise in the preceding 12 h.

The BIA procedure involved the injection of a continuous sinusoidal current (800 A) with a frequency of 50 kHz. The BIA 101 BIVA PRO instrument (Akern SRL, Pontassieve, Italy) was utilized for all measurements, aligning with the rigorous standards recommended by the European Society for Parenteral and Enteral Nutrition [34].

Parameters such as resistance (Rz) and reactance (Xc) of human tissue were measured through BIA. The same instrument was used to assess body cell mass, fat-free mass, fat mass, total body water, and extracellular water. Specialized software (Bodygram PLUS Software v. 1.0, Akern SRL, Pontassieve, Italy) facilitated the calculation of these parameters based on the obtained Rz and Xc values. The phase angle, derived as the arctangent of the Xc/Rz ratio, was also computed as a crucial metric in the evaluation.

2.5. Training Diary

All participants filled out their daily diary, indicating the type of PA performed and the duration. At the end of each day, they reported the total number of daily steps monitored by their heart rate monitor. The diary was used to motivate patients to be physically active, compare participation in the walking group, and know and quantify the PA performed in addition to the proposed work.

When the training diary was handed over to the participants, they were given all the information on how to fill it in correctly.

2.6. Exercise Protocol

2.6.1. Physical Capacity Assessment Tests

Three field tests were performed to assess the subjects' basic conditions and establish the most appropriate intensity of the training program. These included cardiorespiratory capacity, evaluated with the 2 km walk test [35], and strength and flexibility, assessed with the Hand Grip and Sit and Reach tests [36,37]. Subjects performed these tests at the beginning of the project and the end of the three months.

The week before the field tests (3 sessions of 60 min), the participants were adequately instructed on how to carry out the tests correctly so that the results would be as reliable as possible. In these 3 preliminary sessions, the experts explained the correct walking technique and corrected any problems, sensitized the participants on using suitable technical shoes to avoid injuries, and ensured each heart rate monitor functioned correctly and answered any questions.

As far as possible, the tests were reproduced under the same conditions: (a) in the same place, (b) supervised by the same operators, (c) at the same time, and (d) monitored with the same instruments.

2.6.2. Exercise Intervention

PA, organized in "Walking Groups", was structured as follows:

- Frequency. The aerobic exercise was performed outdoors on an urban route thrice a week, on non-consecutive days, for 12 weeks.
- Intensity. The aerobic exercise intensity was moderate (60/75% of HR max); it was monitored through the heart rate monitor and was personalized through Tanaka's

formula [38]. In addition, the Talk Test [39] and the Borg scale [40] were used to measure the rhythm and the perception of fatigue, respectively.
- Type. The aerobic exercise type was walking, ranging from 5 to 10 km/h.
- Time. Each walk had a duration of 60′ for a total of 180′ per week; the single outing lasting 60′ was structured as follows: Warm-up: 5′; Normal walk: 10′; Sustained walking: 30′; Fast walking: 10′; Cool-down: 5′. The entire activity was supervised by experts (Graduates in Preventive and Adapted Physical Activity Science and Techniques), and the presence of the participants at each training session was strictly registered.

2.6.3. Exposure—Global Physical Capacity Score

PC was measured by a series of motor tests of varying difficulty, validated in adult subjects, to assess cardiorespiratory capacity, strength, and flexibility. A PC score was then calculated using the results of each test. Each physical test was scored from 0 to 2 using performance categories (e.g., performance above average = 2 points, average = 1 point, below average or unable to complete the test = 0 points). Then, the scores of the 3 tests were added to obtain an overall physical ability score (possible range of scores between 0 and 6 points). The GPCS used in the present study was adapted from the approach previously proposed by Bouchard et al. [41]. An advantage of calculating and using GPCS is that it provides an overall measure of physical performance that considers several tasks related to daily activities, unlike each test taken individually.

2.7. Outcome Assessment—IBS Severity Scoring System (IBS-SSS)

To assess the GI symptom profile, the GSRS and the IBS-SSS questionnaires were administered. The first is The GSRS is a disease-specific instrument of 15 items combined into five symptom clusters depicting "Reflux", "Abdominal pain", "Indigestion", "Diarrhea", and "Constipation". The GSRS has a seven-point Likert-type scale where 1 represents the absence of troublesome symptoms, and 7 represents very troubling symptoms. The latter is a validated questionnaire that consists of five items with a score ranging from 0 to 500: "Abdominal pain intensity", "Abdominal pain frequency", "Abdominal distension", "Dissatisfaction with bowel habit", and "Interference on life in general". The applied cut-off score to determine the IBS severity was as follows; >75–175 for "mild IBS", 175–300 for "moderate IBS", and >300 for "severe IBS" [42].

2.8. Statistical Analysis

Patients' characteristics were described by mean ± SD (or median values where necessary) and frequency (%) for continuous and categorical variables. For continuous data, the Kruskal–Wallis with Dunn's post-test was used to assess differences among the groups (No IBS subjects, IBS patients pre- and after treatment). The Wilcoxon test was performed to evaluate the effects of treatment on the single variables in IBS patients. Chi-square tests were used to compare categorical data (e.g., results from the 2Km Walking Test, Sit and Reach Test, Hand-Grip Test, and IPAQ). The main outcome is by an ordered logistic regression. As there were two repeated measurements of the outcome, we performed a mixed ordinal logistic model to account for the study's design and the data's correlation structure. After fitting the ordinal logistic model, we obtained predictions (probabilities) using post-estimation tools. The statistical analysis was performed with Stata Statistical Software 18 (Corp, 4905 Lakeway Drive, College Station, TX, USA). The analyses were conducted using RStudio ("Prairie Trillium" Release) for the graphics.

3. Results

The study involved 78 participants, with 40 identified as IBS patients. The No IBS group comprised 38 individuals without lower gut symptoms but experiencing mild symptoms of upper gut diseases, such as dyspepsia or gastroesophageal reflux. The study flow is depicted in Figure 2. All participants adhered to the same exercise program.

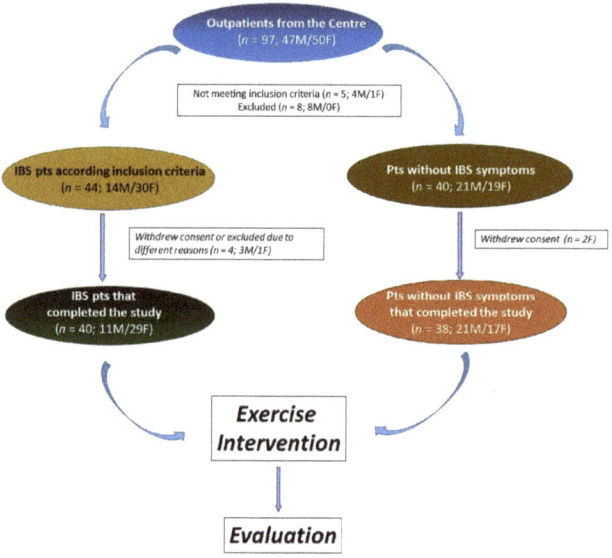

Figure 2. The flowchart of the study.

3.1. Patient Characteristics

The participants' characteristics are shown in Table 1. Comparing the three groups, there were no significant differences regarding anthropometric parameters expressed as BMI, waist and hip circumferences, and waist/hip ratio. As for BIA parameters, the No IBS subjects had slightly but significantly, higher mean values of BCM, FFM, and TBW than IBS subjects, indicating better health and nutritional conditions and hydration status. Furthermore, these parameters remained unchanged at the end of the exercise program in subjects with IBS. Conversely, the GPCS after the PA program was significantly higher ($p < 0.05$) than No IBS subjects and IBS patients before treatment.

Table 1. Characteristics of participants.

		Exercise Intervention		
	No IBS (n.38)	IBS Pre (n. 40)	IBS Post (40)	p
Sex (male/female)	21M/17F	11M/29F		
Age (years)	53.71 ± 7.27	52.10 ± 7.72		
Body mass index	29.96 ± 5.84 [a]	29.04 ± 5.12 [a]	28.80 ± 5.15 [a]	0.0690
Waist circumference	98.69 ± 13.71 [a]	93.04 ± 13.41 [a]	92.71 ± 13.62 [a]	0.1149
Hip circumference	106.53 ± 11.26 [a]	106.22 ± 10.07 [a]	105.51 ± 10.07 [a]	0.0465
Waist/hip ratio	0.93 ± 0.11 [a]	0.87 ± 0.12 [a]	0.88 ± 0.12 [a]	0.0899
PhA (degrees)	6.76 ± 1.06 [a]	6.46 ± 1.07 [a]	6.44 ± 0.98 [a]	0.3671
BCM (kg)	32.51 ± 7.22 [a]	28.90 ± 7.04 [b]	28.62 ± 6.6 [b]	0.0380
FM (kg)	27.82 ± 12.10 [a]	27.21 ± 10.84 [a]	26.72 ± 10.91 [a]	0.9734
FFM (kg)	56.70 ± 10.14 [a]	51.60 ± 9.29 [b]	51.22 ± 8.88 [b]	0.0292
TBW (liters)	41.32 ± 7.68 [a]	37.60 ± 6.84 [b]	37.33 ± 6.44 [b]	0.0340
ECW (liters)	17.57 ± 3.35 [a]	16.44 ± 2.64 [a]	16.36 ± 2.51 [a]	0.2289
Global Physical Capacity Score	2.21 ± 1.76 [a]	2.40 ± 1.53 [a]	3.32 ± 1.68 [b]	<0.0001
IBS scores				
Abdominal pain intensity	1.84 ± 6.62 [a]	24.50 ± 27.26 [b]	12.58 ± 21.92 [b]	<0.0001
Abdominal pain frequency	1.58 ± 5.94 [a]	21.75 ± 29.86 [b]	8.62 ± 18.15 [b]	0.0003
Abdominal Distension	9.21 ± 14.36 [a]	45.75 ± 23.95 [b]	27.80 ± 21.37 [c]	<0.0001
Dissatisfaction with bowel habits	10.39 ± 12.81 [a]	47.75 ± 32.20 [b]	31.25 ± 23.88 [b]	0.0002
Interference on life in general	5.39 ± 9.96 [a]	43.38 ± 25.68 [b]	31.50 ± 27.20 [b]	0.0077
Total score	28.45 ± 26.02 [a]	183.10 ± 79.43 [b]	111.80 ± 76.84 [c]	<0.0001

Table 1. Cont.

	Exercise Intervention			
	No IBS (n.38)	IBS Pre (n. 40)	IBS Post (40)	p
2Km Walking Test				p *
Under the mean	20 (52.6%)	21 (52.5%)	11 (27.5%)	
In mean	16 (42.1%)	15 (37.5%)	20 (50%)	0.0516
Above the mean	2 (5.3%)	4 (10.0%)	9 (22.5%)	
Sit and Reach Test				
Under the mean	23 (60.5%)	22 (55.0%)	16 (40%)	
In mean	2 (5.3%)	4 (10.0%)	4 (10%)	0.4907
Above the mean	13 (34.2%)	14 (35.0%)	20 (50%)	
Hand-Grip Test				
Under the mean	14 (36.8%)	12 (30.0%)	9 (22.5%)	
In mean	12 (31.6%)	15 (37.5%)	11 (27.5%)	0.3771
Above the mean	12 (31.6%)	13 (32.5%)	20 (50%)	
IPAQ Categories °				
<700		13 (34.2%)	11 (27.5%)	
700–2519		19 (50.0%)	19 (47.5%)	0.5723
≥2520		6 (15.8%)	10 (25.0%)	

BMI: body mass index; PhA: phase angle; BCM: body cell mass; FM: fat mass; FFM: fat-free mass; TBW: total body water; ECW: extracellular water. IPAQ: International Physical Activity Questionnaire. Continuous data reported as mean ± SD. Categorical data represented as numbers and percentages. At the Kruskal–Wallis with Dunn's post-test, different letters differ significantly. p: significance obtained by Wilcoxon rank sum test. p *: Significance obtained with the chi-square test. °: IPAQ categories expressed in MET (metabolic equivalent of task). Different superscript letters differ significantly at the Kruskal–Wallis, with Dunn's post-test used.

The results from the IBS-SSS questionnaire indicated a clear difference between IBS patients and No IBS subjects at baseline, as expected. Considering the IBS-SSS items after the programmed exercise, a marked and significant reduction ($p < 0.01$) in single and total items was found. Moreover, the mean total IBS-SSS score changed from moderate to mild after the programmed exercise. The temporal trend of GPCS and IBS-SSS scores and some anthropometric data (GPCS and IBS-SSS scores, BMI, waist circumference, and hip circumference) during intervention time are reported in Appendix A.

Concerning the scores of the 2Km Walking Test, Sit and Reach Test, Hand-Grip Test, and IPAQ, there were no significant differences among the groups.

3.2. Modifications in IBS Categories Based on IBS-SSS and GPCS

Figure 3 illustrates changes in IBS categories based on IBS-SSS score and GPCS after 90 days of treatment.

The aerobic exercise led to 30% (n = 6) of initially "Mild IBS" and 23.5% (n = 4) of "Moderate IBS" subjects transitioning to "Absent IBS symptoms".

Within "Moderate IBS", all but one (70.5% or n = 12) experienced symptom reduction, now classified as "Mild IBS." One person with "Severe IBS" improved to "Mild IBS", resulting in a 60% increase in that category. GPCS showed a 43.5% decrease in "Below average" subjects and doubled the "Above average" number, increasing from 3 to 11 individuals.

The multivariable ordered logistic mixed model (Table 2), which included age (gender, BMI, waist and hip circumference, and IBS severity categories), showed the odds ratio for the highest GPCS category (above the mean) to be 0.04. Subjects above the mean GPCS at the end of the intervention (score of 5 to 6) significantly reduced IBS symptoms and were less likely to develop the same symptoms. Furthermore, the higher the fitness score, the more protective effect of the intervention was on IBS symptoms.

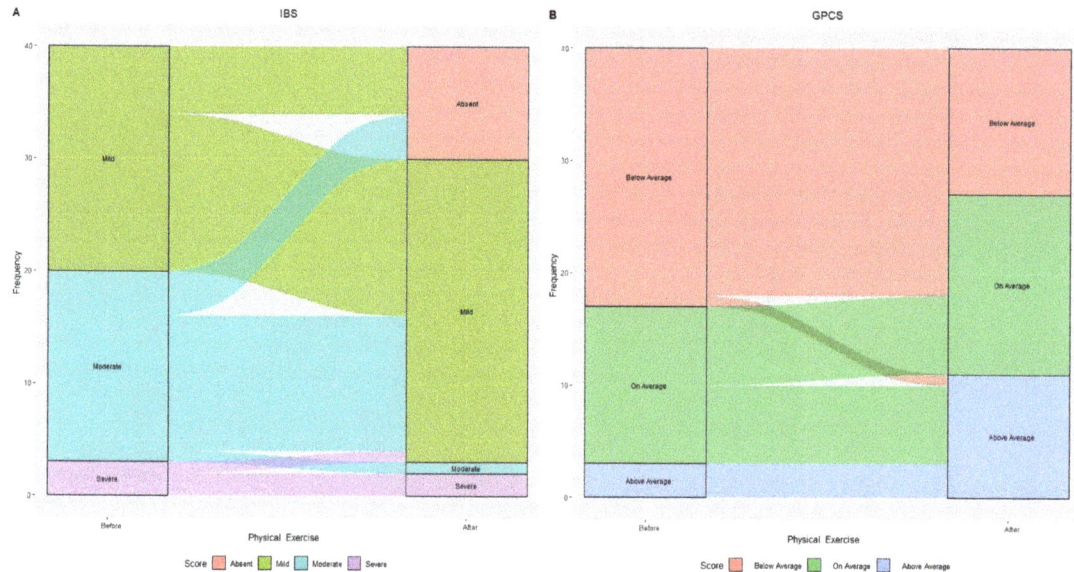

Figure 3. Alluvial plot showing patient flow in relation to IBS categories: "Mild", "Moderate", and "Severe" (**A**) and Global Physical Capacity score (GPCS): "Below Average", "On average", and "Above Average" (**B**) before and after physical exercise.

Table 2. Multilevel mixed-effects ordered logistic regression: effect of physical capacity on irritable bowel syndrome (IBS) severity.

GPCS	Odds Ratio	p-Value	95% CI
Below the mean	1.00		
In mean	0.32	0.10	[0.08, 1.27]
Above the mean	0.04	0.00	[0.00, 0.31]

Adjusted for age, sex, BMI, waist and hip circumference, and IBS categories. GPCS: Global Physical Capacity Score; var (subjects): estimated variance of subjects. var (subjects) 8.28 [3.37, 20.34].

4. Discussion

Present findings show that increasing PA and improving PC could reduce the IBS symptoms, highlighting the positive effects of a structured and controlled aerobic activity intervention lasting 90 days, three times a week (180 min). As expected, 3 months of PA significantly affected the IBS symptom profile. As reported by the IBS-SSS, the total score significantly reduced by 39% compared to baseline, and the same occurred for the Abdominal Distension. In addition, we observed that subjects with an "above average" value in the GPCS had a more significant effect in reducing IBS symptoms than the other categories of the GPCS (namely, "below average" and "average").

There is well-established evidence supporting the health benefits of PA, making it a common recommendation for health promotion and prevention [43]. Regular participation in PA reduces the risk of premature mortality and the development of over 25 chronic medical conditions [43]. Most international PA guidelines for healthy individuals and clinical populations recommend a minimum of 150 min per week of moderate to vigorous intensity PA (MVPA) [44]. Studies have reported that individuals meeting or exceeding international recommendations experienced a 20–30% reduction in the risk of premature mortality and chronic diseases [43].

In this framework, greater risk reductions were observed when objective measurements of health-related PC were utilized [43]. Monitoring PC through validated and accurate tests provides reliable information about the proposed exercise intervention, the improvements achieved by each individual, and the possibility of modifying the program if necessary. Our study utilized a summary score of different field tests (GPCS) to investigate the hypothesized association between improved PC and reduced IBS symptoms. Present findings demonstrated that improved IBS symptoms were effectively accompanied by increased GPCS, which resulted from higher cardiorespiratory capacity, muscle mass, strength, endurance, and flexibility through the exercise program.

Currently, limited and conflicting data are available regarding the association between PA and IBS. While there is evidence of health benefits from moderate exercise in patients with inflammatory bowel disease or functional GI disorders, the safety of more intense exercise has not been clearly established [45].

Controlled and moderate PA has been consistently linked to many health benefits, including improving gastrointestinal (GI) symptoms. While the precise physiological mechanisms remain not entirely elucidated, several factors contribute to this positive relationship.

One significant contributor is the enhancement of gut motility achieved through increased bowel contractions and reduced transit time [46]. This heightened motility can positively impact digestion and overall GI function. Additionally, controlled PA fosters improved blood flow, promoting the GI tract's health. The positive effects extend to the modulation of inflammation through anti-inflammatory mechanisms, further contributing to GI well-being [46].

PA plays a role in stress reduction through cortisol regulation, which has implications for GI health, given the well-established link between stress and gastrointestinal symptoms. Moreover, there is evidence of positive effects on gut microbiota diversity, with regular exercise potentially influencing the composition and function of the microbial community in the digestive system [47].

Hormonal regulation is another key aspect, with controlled PA potentially leading to the release of glucagon-like peptide-1 (GLP-1), which is associated with improved gut function. Weight management is also crucial, as PA can aid in preventing obesity-related GI issues [48].

Furthermore, the positive impact of moderate PA extends to enhanced immune function, which plays a vital role in overall GI health [49]. Finally, the mind–body connection is a holistic aspect that influences psychological well-being, positively impacting GI health overall [50].

It is important to note that individual responses to PA may vary significantly among individuals, highlighting the need for personalized approaches to understanding and harnessing the GI benefits of controlled and moderate PA.

Indeed, some previous studies have reported that moderate PA improves IBS symptoms. On the other hand, a systematic review evidenced that increasing exercise intensity and duration can paradoxically lead to intestinal damage, increased permeability, endotoxemia, impaired gastric emptying, slowed small intestinal transit, and malabsorption. Significant GI disturbances occur with exercise stress lasting ≥ 2 h at 60% VO2 max, regardless of the fitness status [51]. Furthermore, case–control studies have shown lower levels of PA in patients with IBS, while other researchers have found no significant association between PA and IBS. In this context, Omagari et al. [51] reported a high level of PA among patients with IBS compared to those without IBS.

Interestingly, our study on IBS patients from Southern Italy did not find a substantial difference in PA levels at baseline between patients and No IBS subjects. This was probably related to the fact that the IBS group consisted mainly of patients with mild and moderate IBS, according to the classification based on the IBS-SSS questionnaire. However, after evaluation through field tests, we observed lower PC in No IBS subjects compared to those with IBS, in agreement with previously reported findings [20].

Further studies are surely needed to clarify this link. Our results again support the recommendation to increase PA in subjects with IBS and confirm previous findings indicating a protective effect of PA on GI symptoms [20,52].

Although PA should be recommended for patients with IBS, as suggested in the literature [22,53], limited studies provide precise guidance on the exercise program with specific FITT principles (frequency, intensity, time, and type).

The current findings highlight the importance of objectively monitoring participants' physical capabilities to implement effective interventions. A three-month moderate-intensity walking regimen, performed thrice weekly, yielded several advantages, especially for IBS patients. As measured by GPCS, augmented PC resulted in a significant reduction in IBS symptoms in this cohort. The study indicates that achieving an "above the average" score is crucial for eliciting statistically significant outcomes, making GPCS a valuable prognostic tool for personalized treatment criteria.

Interestingly, the adherence of the walking group to the program was total in our study, attributed to the enjoyment participants experienced during the exercise [54]. Indeed, it is well known that walking groups are successful both in contributing to the improvement of participants' health and well-being and in attracting a large number of people at the same time, with low levels of drop-out [55]. Furthermore, the benefits of this type of training were evidenced by the participant's willingness to continue walking even after the project was completed, so the exercise intervention was not just an end but the start of a change in the participants' lifestyle.

Some methodological issues need to be considered. The program's main strength was its supervised nature by trained personnel. Despite the relatively small number of participants per group, three trainers were assigned to each session to establish a personalized connection with each participant, resulting in full program adherence. The training protocol was meticulously designed, adhering to the FITT principles' specific parameters and guidelines established by major international associations [56]. The exercise prescription was provided from a dose–response perspective to achieve the best results for individuals with IBS. Moreover, the presented results possess practical clinical applications and do not necessitate costly resources.

Further studies could be useful for advancing our knowledge about the relationship between physical exercise and IBS by exploring a broader range of activities and refining the prescription process for better, more personalized outcomes. This approach could have the potential to contribute significantly to the development of effective and individualized interventions for managing IBS symptoms through PA.

Nevertheless, certain limitations should be acknowledged. Although the GPCS has been utilized in prior studies, it needs formal validation. However, this score relies on three tests widely recognized in the literature for measuring physical capabilities. These tests are validated, repeatable, reproducible, and objective. Additionally, the small sample size may only represent a subset of the IBS population. Nevertheless, similar studies have shown that a comparable sample size was sufficient to detect significant differences in PA exposure.

5. Conclusions

Moderate-intensity aerobic exercise, performed for at least 180 min per week, can improve GI symptoms in patients with IBS and should, therefore, be added to the list of recommended primary interventions for patients with IBS. Additionally, monitoring the GPCS of IBS patients offers valuable insights into the correlation between PA and symptom severity. Through continuous PC monitoring, healthcare professionals can evaluate the impact of exercise and lifestyle modifications on the overall well-being of these patients. This assessment may reveal improvements in bowel habits, reduced pain levels, and an enhanced quality of life. Furthermore, regular monitoring allows healthcare professionals to tailor treatment plans and interventions more effectively, addressing specific symptoms and optimizing outcomes for patients with IBS.

Author Contributions: Conceptualization, A.B., F.R. and A.R.O.; data curation, I.F., R.C. and L.P.; formal analysis, A.B., F.R., R.D., C.B. and A.R.O.; investigation, I.F., R.C., B.D., A.I. and A.C.; writing—original draft, A.B., F.R. and A.R.O.; writing—review and editing, A.B., F.R., G.R., L.P., B.D., A.I., A.C. and A.R.O. All authors have read and agreed to the published version of the manuscript.

Funding: This research was funded by the Italian Ministry of Health RC 2023, Prog. N°16 (D.D.G. n. 66/22).

Institutional Review Board Statement: The study was conducted in accordance with the Declaration of Helsinki and approved by the Institutional Ethics Committees of IRCCS Ospedale Oncologico—Istituto Tumori Giovanni Paolo II, Bari, Italy, prot. N. 177/EC of date 13 May 2022.

Informed Consent Statement: Informed consent was obtained from all subjects involved in the study.

Data Availability Statement: Data are available upon reasonable request.

Conflicts of Interest: The authors declare no conflict of interest.

Appendix A

Table A1. Temporal trend of GPCS and IBS-SSS scores and some anthropometrical data during intervention time.

	No IBS Exercise Intervention	
	PRE	POST
N.	21M/17F	21M/17F
GPCS	2.21 ± 1.76	3.13 ± 1.88
IBS-SSS	28.45 ± 26.02	22.26 ± 28.78
BMI	29.96 ± 5.84	29.47 ± 5.45
WC	98.69 ± 13.71	96.32 ± 11.19
HC	106.53 ± 11.26	106.27 ± 10.02

N: number of subjects; GPCS: Global Physical Capacity Score; IBS-SSS: IBS Severity Scoring System; BMI: Body Mass Index; WC: Waist Circumference; HC: Hip Circumference. Data are reported as mean ± SD.

References

1. Vandvik, P.O.; Lydersen, S.; Farup, P.G. Prevalence, comorbidity and impact of irritable bowel syndrome in Norway. *Scand. J. Gastroenterol.* **2006**, *41*, 650–656. [CrossRef]
2. Wilson, S.; Roberts, L.; Roalfe, A.; Bridge, P.; Singh, S. Prevalence of irritable bowel syndrome: A community survey. *Br. J. Gen. Pract.* **2004**, *54*, 495–502.
3. Thompson, W.G.; Longstreth, G.; Drossman, D.; Heaton, K.; Irvine, E.; Müller-Lissner, S. Functional bowel disorders and functional abdominal pain. *Gut* **1999**, *45*, II43–II47. [CrossRef] [PubMed]
4. Kearney, D.J.; Brown-Chang, J. Complementary and alternative medicine for IBS in adults: Mind–body interventions. *Nat. Clin. Pract. Gastroenterol. Hepatol.* **2008**, *5*, 624–636. [CrossRef]
5. Spanier, J.A.; Howden, C.W.; Jones, M.P. A systematic review of alternative therapies in the irritable bowel syndrome. *Arch. Intern. Med.* **2003**, *163*, 265–274. [CrossRef] [PubMed]
6. Wald, A.; Rakel, D. Behavioral and complementary approaches for the treatment of irritable bowel syndrome. *Nutr. Clin. Pract.* **2008**, *23*, 284–292. [CrossRef] [PubMed]
7. Wu, J.C. Complementary and alternative medicine modalities for the treatment of irritable bowel syndrome: Facts or myths? *Gastroenterol. Hepatol.* **2010**, *6*, 705.
8. Cozma-Petruţ, A.; Loghin, F.; Miere, D.; Dumitraşcu, D.L. Diet in irritable bowel syndrome: What to recommend, not what to forbid to patients! *World J. Gastroenterol.* **2017**, *23*, 3771. [CrossRef]
9. Ooi, S.L.; Correa, D.; Pak, S.C. Probiotics, prebiotics, and low FODMAP diet for irritable bowel syndrome–What is the current evidence? *Complement. Ther. Med.* **2019**, *43*, 73–80. [CrossRef] [PubMed]
10. Orlando, A.; Tutino, V.; Notarnicola, M.; Riezzo, G.; Linsalata, M.; Clemente, C.; Prospero, L.; Martulli, M.; D'Attoma, B.; De Nunzio, V. Improved symptom profiles and minimal inflammation in IBS-D patients undergoing a long-term low-FODMAP diet: A lipidomic perspective. *Nutrients* **2020**, *12*, 1652. [CrossRef]
11. Riezzo, G.; Prospero, L.; Orlando, A.; Linsalata, M.; D'Attoma, B.; Ignazzi, A.; Giannelli, G.; Russo, F. A Tritordeum-Based Diet for Female Patients with Diarrhea-Predominant Irritable Bowel Syndrome: Effects on Abdominal Bloating and Psychological Symptoms. *Nutrients* **2023**, *15*, 1361. [CrossRef] [PubMed]

12. Blumenthal, J.A.; Babyak, M.A.; Doraiswamy, P.M.; Watkins, L.; Hoffman, B.M.; Barbour, K.A.; Herman, S.; Craighead, W.E.; Brosse, A.L.; Waugh, R. Exercise and pharmacotherapy in the treatment of major depressive disorder. *Psychosom. Med.* **2007**, *69*, 587. [CrossRef]
13. Mannerkorpi, K. Exercise in fibromyalgia. *Curr. Opin. Rheumatol.* **2005**, *17*, 190–194. [CrossRef]
14. Steindorf, K.; Jedrychowski, W.; Schmidt, M.; Popiela, T.; Penar, A.; Galas, A.; Wahrendorf, J. Case-control study of lifetime occupational and recreational physical activity and risks of colon and rectal cancer. *Eur. J. Cancer Prev.* **2005**, *14*, 363–371. [CrossRef] [PubMed]
15. Wolin, K.Y.; Lee, I.M.; Colditz, G.A.; Glynn, R.J.; Fuchs, C.; Giovannucci, E. Leisure-time physical activity patterns and risk of colon cancer in women. *Int. J. Cancer* **2007**, *121*, 2776–2781. [CrossRef] [PubMed]
16. Zhou, C.; Zhao, E.; Li, Y.; Jia, Y.; Li, F. Exercise therapy of patients with irritable bowel syndrome: A systematic review of randomized controlled trials. *Neurogastroenterol. Motil.* **2019**, *31*, e13461. [CrossRef]
17. Costantino, A.; Pessarelli, T.; Vecchiato, M.; Vecchi, M.; Basilisco, G.; Ermolao, A. A practical guide to the proper prescription of physical activity in patients with irritable bowel syndrome. *Dig. Liver Dis.* **2022**, *54*, 1600–1604. [CrossRef] [PubMed]
18. Belvederi Murri, M.; Folesani, F.; Zerbinati, L.; Nanni, M.G.; Ounalli, H.; Caruso, R.; Grassi, L. Physical activity promotes health and reduces cardiovascular mortality in depressed populations: A literature overview. *Int. J. Environ. Res. Public Health* **2020**, *17*, 5545. [CrossRef]
19. Villoria, A.; Serra, J.; Azpiroz, F.; Malagelada, J.-R. Physical activity and intestinal gas clearance in patients with bloating. *Off. J. Am. Coll. Gastroenterol. ACG* **2006**, *101*, 2552–2557. [CrossRef]
20. Dainese, R.; Serra, J.; Azpiroz, F.; Malagelada, J.-R. Effects of physical activity on intestinal gas transit and evacuation in healthy subjects. *Am. J. Med.* **2004**, *116*, 536–539. [CrossRef] [PubMed]
21. Johannesson, E.; Ringström, G.; Abrahamsson, H.; Sadik, R. Intervention to increase physical activity in irritable bowel syndrome shows long-term positive effects. *World J. Gastroenterol. WJG* **2015**, *21*, 600. [CrossRef] [PubMed]
22. Johannesson, E.; Simrén, M.; Strid, H.; Bajor, A.; Sadik, R. Physical activity improves symptoms in irritable bowel syndrome: A randomized controlled trial. *Off. J. Am. Coll. Gastroenterol. ACG* **2011**, *106*, 915–922. [CrossRef]
23. Physical Activity Guidelines Advisory Committee. *Physical Activity Guidelines Advisory Committee Report*; US Department of Health and Human Services: Washington, DC, USA, 2008; A1-H14.
24. Lee, I.-M.; Skerrett, P.J. Physical activity and all-cause mortality: What is the dose-response relation? *Med. Sci. Sports Exerc.* **2001**, *33*, S459–S471. [CrossRef] [PubMed]
25. Murphy, M.H.; Nevill, A.M.; Murtagh, E.M.; Holder, R.L. The effect of walking on fitness, fatness and resting blood pressure: A meta-analysis of randomised, controlled trials. *Prev. Med.* **2007**, *44*, 377–385. [CrossRef]
26. Hu, F.B.; Sigal, R.J.; Rich-Edwards, J.W.; Colditz, G.A.; Solomon, C.G.; Willett, W.C.; Speizer, F.E.; Manson, J.E. Walking compared with vigorous physical activity and risk of type 2 diabetes in women: A prospective study. *JAMA* **1999**, *282*, 1433–1439. [CrossRef]
27. Fox, K. *At Least Five a Week: Evidence on the Impact of Physical Activity and Its Relationship to Health—A Report from the Chief Medical Officer*; Senior Scientific Editor for Department of Health: London, UK, 2004.
28. MIND. *The MIND Guide to Physical Activity*; MIND: London, UK, 2008.
29. Kwak, L.; Kremers, S.; Walsh, A.; Brug, H. How is your walking group running? *Health Educ.* **2006**, *106*, 21–31. [CrossRef]
30. Doughty, K. Walking together: The embodied and mobile production of a therapeutic landscape. *Health Place* **2013**, *24*, 140–146. [CrossRef] [PubMed]
31. Pate, R.R. A new definition of youth fitness. *Physician Sportsmed.* **1983**, *11*, 77–83. [CrossRef]
32. Caspersen, C.J.; Powell, K.E.; Christenson, G.M. Physical activity, exercise, and physical fitness: Definitions and distinctions for health-related research. *Public Health Rep.* **1985**, *100*, 126.
33. Lee, P.H.; Macfarlane, D.J.; Lam, T.H.; Stewart, S.M. Validity of the international physical activity questionnaire short form (IPAQ-SF): A systematic review. *Int. J. Behav. Nutr. Phys. Act.* **2011**, *8*, 115. [CrossRef]
34. Khalil, S.F.; Mohktar, M.S.; Ibrahim, F. The theory and fundamentals of bioimpedance analysis in clinical status monitoring and diagnosis of diseases. *Sensors* **2014**, *14*, 10895–10928. [CrossRef] [PubMed]
35. Laukkanen, R.; Oja, P.; Pasanen, M.; Vuori, I. Validity of a two kilometre walking test for estimating maximal aerobic power in overweight adults. *Int. J. Obes. Relat. Metab. Disord. J. Int. Assoc. Study Obes.* **1992**, *16*, 263–268.
36. Pearn, J.; Bullock, K. A portable hand-grip dynamometer. *J. Paediatr. Child Health* **1979**, *15*, 107–109. [CrossRef] [PubMed]
37. Hoeger, W.W.; Hopkins, D.R. A comparison of the sit and reach and the modified sit and reach in the measurement of flexibility in women. *Res. Q. Exerc. Sport* **1992**, *63*, 191–195. [CrossRef] [PubMed]
38. Tanaka, H.; Monahan, K.D.; Seals, D.R. Age-predicted maximal heart rate revisited. *J. Am. Coll. Cardiol.* **2001**, *37*, 153–156. [CrossRef]
39. Foster, C.; Porcari, J.P.; Anderson, J.; Paulson, M.; Smaczny, D.; Webber, H.; Doberstein, S.T.; Udermann, B. The talk test as a marker of exercise training intensity. *J. Cardiopulm. Rehabil. Prev.* **2008**, *28*, 24–30. [CrossRef]
40. Wilson, R.C.; Jones, P. A comparison of the visual analogue scale and modified Borg scale for the measurement of dyspnoea during exercise. *Clin. Sci.* **1989**, *76*, 277–282. [CrossRef]
41. Bouchard, D.R.; Soucy, L.; Sénéchal, M.; Dionne, I.J.; Brochu, M. Impact of resistance training with or without caloric restriction on physical capacity in obese older women. *Menopause* **2009**, *16*, 66–72. [CrossRef]

42. Francis, C.Y.; Morris, J.; Whorwell, P.J. The irritable bowel severity scoring system: A simple method of monitoring irritable bowel syndrome and its progress. *Aliment. Pharmacol. Ther.* **1997**, *11*, 395–402. [CrossRef]
43. Warburton, D.E.; Bredin, S.S. Health benefits of physical activity: A systematic review of current systematic reviews. *Curr. Opin. Cardiol.* **2017**, *32*, 541–556. [CrossRef]
44. Warburton, D.E.; Charlesworth, S.; Ivey, A.; Nettlefold, L.; Bredin, S.S. A systematic review of the evidence for Canada's Physical Activity Guidelines for Adults. *Int. J. Behav. Nutr. Phys. Act.* **2010**, *7*, 39. [CrossRef]
45. Costa, R.; Snipe, R.; Kitic, C.; Gibson, P. Systematic review: Exercise-induced gastrointestinal syndrome—Implications for health and intestinal disease. *Aliment. Pharmacol. Ther.* **2017**, *46*, 246–265. [CrossRef] [PubMed]
46. Peters, H.P.; De Vries, W.R.; Vanberge-Henegouwen, G.P.; Akkermans, L.M. Potential benefits and hazards of physical activity and exercise on the gastrointestinal tract. *Gut* **2001**, *48*, 435–439. [CrossRef] [PubMed]
47. Monda, V.; Villano, I.; Messina, A.; Valenzano, A.; Esposito, T.; Moscatelli, F.; Viggiano, A.; Cibelli, G.; Chieffi, S.; Monda, M.; et al. Exercise Modifies the Gut Microbiota with Positive Health Effects. *Oxidative Med. Cell. Longev.* **2017**, *2017*, 3831972. [CrossRef]
48. Madsbad, S. The role of glucagon-like peptide-1 impairment in obesity and potential therapeutic implications. *Diabetes Obes. Metab.* **2014**, *16*, 9–21. [CrossRef]
49. Nieman, D.C.; Wentz, L.M. The compelling link between physical activity and the body's defense system. *J. Sport Health Sci.* **2019**, *8*, 201–217. [CrossRef]
50. Caes, L.; Orchard, A.; Christie, D. Connecting the mind–body split: Understanding the relationship between symptoms and emotional well-being in chronic pain and functional gastrointestinal disorders. *Healthcare* **2017**, *5*, 93. [CrossRef]
51. Omagari, K.; Murayama, T.; Tanaka, Y.; Yoshikawa, C.; Inoue, S.-i.; Ichimura, M.; Hatanaka, M.; Saimei, M.; Muto, K.; Tobina, T. Mental, physical, dietary, and nutritional effects on irritable bowel syndrome in young Japanese women. *Intern. Med.* **2013**, *52*, 1295–1301. [CrossRef]
52. De Schryver, A.M.; Keulemans, Y.C.; Peters, H.P.; Akkermans, L.M.; Smout, A.J.; De Vries, W.R.; Van Berge-Henegouwen, G.P. Effects of regular physical activity on defecation pattern in middle-aged patients complaining of chronic constipation. *Scand. J. Gastroenterol.* **2005**, *40*, 422–429. [CrossRef] [PubMed]
53. Colwell, L.; Prather, C.; Phillips, S.; Zinsmeister, A. Effects of an irritable bowel syndrome educational class on health-promoting behaviors and symptoms. *Am. J. Gastroenterol.* **1998**, *93*, 901–905. [CrossRef] [PubMed]
54. Parfitt, G.; Hughes, S. The exercise intensity–affect relationship: Evidence and implications for exercise behavior. *J. Exerc. Sci. Fit.* **2009**, *7*, S34–S41. [CrossRef]
55. Hanson, S.; Jones, A. Is there evidence that walking groups have health benefits? A systematic review and meta-analysis. *Br. J. Sports Med.* **2015**, *49*, 710–715. [CrossRef] [PubMed]
56. Thompson, P.D.; Arena, R.; Riebe, D.; Pescatello, L.S. ACSM's new preparticipation health screening recommendations from ACSM's guidelines for exercise testing and prescription. *Curr. Sports Med. Rep.* **2013**, *12*, 215–217. [CrossRef] [PubMed]

Disclaimer/Publisher's Note: The statements, opinions and data contained in all publications are solely those of the individual author(s) and contributor(s) and not of MDPI and/or the editor(s). MDPI and/or the editor(s) disclaim responsibility for any injury to people or property resulting from any ideas, methods, instructions or products referred to in the content.

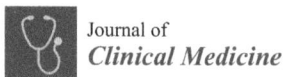

Article

The Influence of Interval Training Combined with Occlusion and Cooling on Selected Indicators of Blood, Muscle Metabolism and Oxidative Stress

Bartłomiej Ptaszek [1,*], Szymon Podsiadło [2], Olga Czerwińska-Ledwig [3], Bartosz Zając [4], Rafał Niżankowski [5], Piotr Mika [2] and Aneta Teległów [3]

1. Institute of Applied Sciences, University of Physical Education in Krakow, 31-571 Krakow, Poland
2. Institute of Clinical Rehabilitation, University of Physical Education in Krakow, 31-571 Krakow, Poland; szymon.podsiadlo@awf.krakow.pl (S.P.); piotr.mika@awf.krakow.pl (P.M.)
3. Institute of Basic Sciences, University of Physical Education in Krakow, 31-571 Krakow, Poland; olga.czerwinska@awf.krakow.pl (O.C.-L.); aneta.teleglow@awf.krakow.pl (A.T.)
4. Laboratory of Functional Diagnostics, Central Scientific and Research Laboratory, University of Physical Education in Krakow, 31-571 Krakow, Poland; bartosz.zajac@awf.krakow.pl
5. Sano Science, Centre for Computational Medicine, 30-054 Krakow, Poland; rtn@wp.pl
* Correspondence: bartlomiej.ptaszek@awf.krakow.pl

Abstract: There is increasing evidence to support the use of interval training and/or low-impact blood flow restriction exercises in musculoskeletal rehabilitation. The aim of the study was to assess the effect of interval training combined with occlusion and cooling in terms of changes in selected blood parameters affecting the development and progression of atherosclerosis of the lower limbs, as well as selected parameters of muscle metabolism and oxidative stress affecting the growth of muscle mass and regeneration after training. Material and methods: The study included 30 young, healthy and untrained people. The VASPER (Vascular Performance) training system was used—High-Intensity Interval Training with the simultaneous use of occlusion and local cryotherapy. Blood from the project participants was collected six times (2 weeks before the start of training, on the day of training, after the first training, after the 10th training, after the 20th training and two weeks after the end of training). The subjects were randomly divided into three groups: exercises only (controlled), with occlusion and with occlusion and local cryotherapy. Results: Statistical analysis of changes in the average values of indicators in all study groups showed a significant change increase due to the time of testing IGF-1 (F = 2.37, $p = 0.04$), XOD (F = 14.26, $p = 0.00$), D-Dimer (F = 2.90, $p = 0.02$), and decrease in MDA (F = 7.14, $p = 0.00$), T-AOC (F = 11.17, $p = 0.00$), PT Quick (F = 26.37, $p = 0.00$), INR (F = 8.79, $p = 0.00$), TT (F = 3.81, $p = 0.00$). The most pronounced changes were observed in the occlusion and cooling group. Conclusions: Both interval training without and with the modifications used in the study influences coagulation and oxidative stress parameters and, to a small extent, muscle metabolism. It seems reasonable to use occlusion and local cryotherapy in combination with occlusion.

Keywords: coagulology; muscle metabolism; oxidative stress; interval training; occlusion; VASPER

Citation: Ptaszek, B.; Podsiadło, S.; Czerwińska-Ledwig, O.; Zając, B.; Niżankowski, R.; Mika, P.; Teległów, A. The Influence of Interval Training Combined with Occlusion and Cooling on Selected Indicators of Blood, Muscle Metabolism and Oxidative Stress. *J. Clin. Med.* **2023**, *12*, 7636. https://doi.org/10.3390/jcm12247636

Academic Editors: Kazuhisa Asai and Yoshiaki Minakata

Received: 5 November 2023
Revised: 7 December 2023
Accepted: 8 December 2023
Published: 12 December 2023

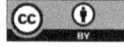

Copyright: © 2023 by the authors. Licensee MDPI, Basel, Switzerland. This article is an open access article distributed under the terms and conditions of the Creative Commons Attribution (CC BY) license (https://creativecommons.org/licenses/by/4.0/).

1. Introduction

Chronic ischemia of the lower limbs is a condition resulting from insufficient supply of oxygen to the tissues of the lower limbs associated with impaired blood flow in the arteries, caused in 97% of cases by atherosclerosis of the lower limbs. The progressive atherosclerotic process causes narrowing and occlusion of the arterial lumen, consequently leading to chronic ischemia of the lower limbs manifested by pain, shortening of walking distance and intermittent claudication [1]. From a clinical point of view, the finding of atherosclerotic lesions in one place means that it is necessary to take into account the possibility of atherosclerosis also in other vascular locations, which may be associated with the risk of heart attacks and strokes [2]. Conservative and pharmacological treatment includes modification of risk factors such as smoking, dyslipidemia, diabetes, and hypertension and is aimed at stopping the progressive atherosclerotic process [2]. An important and decisive role in the effectiveness of treatment is attributed to regular physical activity, which allows the achievement of the best and most long-lasting effects [3]. The beneficial effects of BFR (blood flow restriction) training were popularized in the 1940s in Japan [4].

Numerous studies have shown that BRF training affects muscle strength, endurance and hypertrophy [5–7]. So far, according to the standards of The American College of Sports Medicine, the effective training load that can induce beneficial hypertrophic changes in muscles is 60–100% of 1RM (Rep Max) [5,7]. Recent publications show that this effect can also be achieved by using a low exercise intensity of 20–50% 1RM combined with venous or arterial occlusion, thus avoiding significant damage to muscle fibers [6,8–10]. This mechanism is associated with the increased activation of type II FT (Fast Twitching) muscle fibers in oxygen-limited work conditions [11,12].

The effectiveness of exercises combined with occlusion causes significant changes in the level of muscle oxygenation, an increase in anaerobic metabolism products and a significant endocrine response, visible in changes in selected blood parameters [13]. During exercises with occlusion, more than twice the level of lactic acid concentration is exposed, compared to exercises without occlusion [14]. The increased increase in lactic acid levels persists for up to 10 min after the end of exercise, while after approximately 60 min the concentration is still higher than the initial level before the start of the study [9,15]. BRF training also significantly contributes to increasing the concentration of growth hormone (GH), the highest level of which can be observed 20 min after exercise [11,14,16–18].

GH plays a key role in preventing atherosclerosis and stimulates the production of peptides called insulin-like growth factors (IGF-1 and IGF-2) [11]. GH and IGF-1 are important mitogenic factors for cardiomyocytes [19]. Their deficiency is associated with a reduced heart mass, decreased late diastolic volume and reduced ejection fraction [19]. The observable increase in the level of VEGF (vascular endothelial growth factor) also plays a major role in the process of angiogenesis and the creation of collateral circulation [20]. Metabolic changes occurring in response to BRF exercises are an important factor influencing the increase in VEGF, which is involved in the process of preventing and developing atherosclerotic lesions.

Pre-cooling of the body applied before training can significantly increase the body's performance and exercise intensity, both increasing the capacity for prolonged training and the intensity of short-term exercise [21,22]. The pre-cooling mechanism related to the constriction of superficial vessels and probably an increase in blood flow in the muscles generates more efficient elimination of metabolites, reducing the level of DOMS (delayed onset muscle soreness) and lowering the heart rate [21,22].

The aim of the study was to assess the effect of interval training combined with occlusion and cooling in terms of changes in selected blood parameters affecting the development and progression of atherosclerosis of the lower limbs, as well as selected parameters of muscle metabolism and oxidative stress affecting the growth of muscle mass and regeneration after training. Physical exercise combined with occlusion and cooling can be implemented and bring tangible benefits among patients with atherosclerosis of the lower limb arteries, but it can also be widely used in the creation of innovative and effective rehabilitation programs, including patients with chronic ischemia of the lower limbs and other diseases. Analysis of changes in indicators can contribute a lot to science in terms of planning effective therapy.

2. Materials and Methods

The research was conducted at the University of Physical Education in Krakow (Poland). The subjects were students who were included in the research program after obtaining medical and physiotherapeutic qualifications. To conduct the experiment, written consent was obtained from the Bioethics Committee at the Regional Medical Chamber in Krakow (164/KBL/OIL/2021). The trials were also registered with the Australian New Zealand Clinical Trials Registry (ACTRN12622000734763). Each volunteer received comprehensive information about the project; if any doubts arose, they had the opportunity to obtain clarification, and then each of them gave informed, written consent to participate in the study (Figure 1). The research covered a group of 30 people, divided into further groups according to the ballot type:

- A total of 10 people performed VASPER Systems LLC (Limited Liability Company) training (Figure 2) without occlusion and cooling (Group CONT)—age [years]: 23.00 ± 0.00; body height [cm]: 164.50 ± 6.44; body mass [kg]: 58.96 ± 10.34.
- A total of 10 people performed VASPER Systems LLC training using occlusion without cooling—the pressure in the occlusion cuffs was 10 mmHg lower than the systolic pressure (Group OCC)—age [years]: 23.22 ± 0.44; body height [cm]: 169.83 ± 9.81; body mass [kg]: 66.31 ± 11.77.
- A total of 10 people performed VASPER Systems LLC training using occlusion and cooling—occlusion as in point 2, additionally combined with activation of the cooling system provided by cuffs and cooling mats located under the feet and in the seat of the subject (Group OCC-COO)—age [years]: 23.25 ± 0.46; body height [cm]: 172.13 ± 9.07; body mass [kg]: 69.45 ± 13.99.

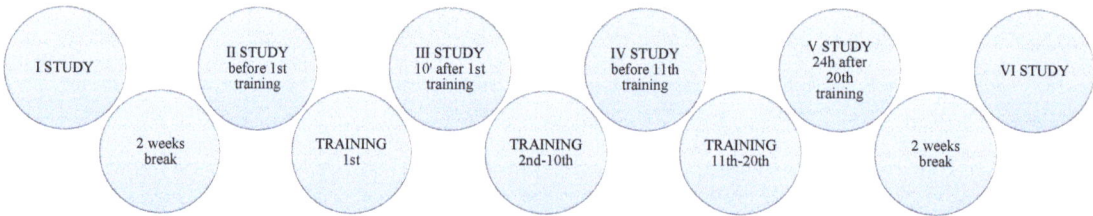

Figure 1. The course of the study.

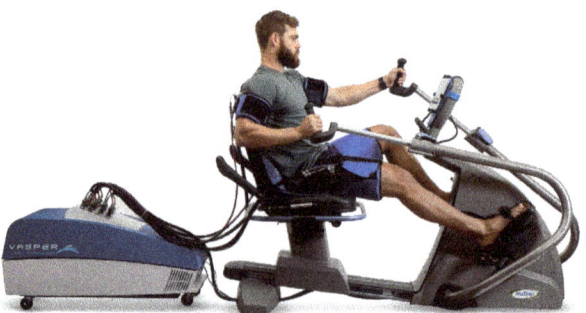

Figure 2. VASPER device (by VASPER Systems LLC).

Inclusion criteria: age 20–25, general good health, no comorbidities, no contraindications to participate in HIIT (High-Intensity Interval Training), not engaging in regular physical training, no changes in diet before or during the research.

2.1. Analysis of Blood Parameters

Blood for the study was collected from fasting subjects (min. 12 h), from the basilic, cephalic or median vein of the elbow, six times (2 weeks before the start of training, on the day of training, after the first training, after the 10th training, after the 20th training and two weeks after the end of training) using vacuum tubes (for serum testing 6 mL) by a qualified laboratory diagnostician in accordance with applicable protocols. aPTT (Activated Partial Thromboplastin Time), Fibrinogen, D-Dimer, TT (Thrombin Time), PT Quick, and INR

(International Normalized Ratio) were determined using the BCS XP analyzer (Siemens Healthcare Diagnostics Product GmbH, Marburg, Germany). CORT (Cortisol) was determined using IMMULITE® 2000 XPi assays (Siemens Healthcare Diagnostics Product GmbH, Marburg, Germany). MIO (Myoglobin) was determined using Alinity™ and STAT Myoglobin Reagent Kit (Abbott, Chicago, IL, USA). HGH (Human Growth Hormone), IGF-1 (Insulin-like Growth Factor 1), VEGF (Vascular Endothelial Growth Factor), MDA (Malondialdehyde), T-AOC (Total Antioxidant Capacity), TOS (Total Oxidative Status) and XOD (Xanthine Oxidase) were determined in the serum. The indices were investigated with photometric tests: HGH—ELISA Kit and IGF-1 600 ELISA Kit (DRG Instruments GmbH, Marburg, Germany); Human VEGF Kit, Human MDA Kit, Human T-AOC Kit, Human TOS Kit, Human XOD Kit (Shanghai Sunred Biological Technology Co., Shanghai, China). The procedure was in accordance with the manufacturer's recommendations.

2.2. Description of the Intervention

Before starting training, each subject underwent an exercise test with lactate measurements (Żołądź Test on the VASPER device), and individual loads not exceeding the lactate threshold were determined. Each participant took part in 20 training sessions (every other day). The training took place at the Functional Diagnostics Laboratory of the University of Physical Education in Krakow.

- OCC-COO group—HIIT training combined with occlusion (on the arms and thighs) and local cooling (built-in cryotherapy system under the feet and under the seat). The pressure in the occlusive cuffs (constant) was 10 mmHg lower than the systolic pressure. The cooling and occlusion system was activated for the entire duration of each training unit. Each session consisted of
    - Introductory part (approx. 2 min)—warm-up, preparation for exercise;
    - Main part (approx. 20 min)—training consisting of 3×6 min and 1 min of rest between intervals;
    - Final part (approx. 2 min)—calming down, conscious muscle relaxation;
- Group OCC—like OCC-COO training, with an occlusion variant, but without cooling;
- CONT group—training as in the previous groups, but without the occlusion and cooling variant.

2.3. Statistical Analysis

Descriptive statistics were determined: mean (x) as well as standard deviation (SD). The normality of distributions was verified with the Shapiro–Wilk test. Comparisons within and between groups were performed using ANOVA for repeated measures. For comparisons between groups, a multivariate ANOVA was used. If significant changes were observed, post hoc tests were performed. The significance level of $p = 0.05$ was adopted in the analyses. In order to determine sample size, the formula for the minimum sample size was used, in which the confidence interval was 95%, the fraction size of 0.5 and the maximum error of 5% were assumed. The analyses were performed with the use of the Statistica 13 package (Tibco Software Inc., Palo Alto, CA, USA).

3. Results

The results are presented in Tables 1–5. Comparisons carried out in individual groups showed statistically significant differences:

- Increase in IGF-1 in the OCC-COO group ($F = 2.85$, $p = 0.03$), XOD in the OCC-COO group ($F = 10.69$, $p = 0.00$), OCC group ($F = 4.42$, $p = 0.00$) and in the CONT group ($F = 6.48$, $p = 0.00$), fibrinogen in the OCC-COO group ($F = 2.81$, $p = 0.03$), and D-Dimer in the OCC-COO group ($F = 2.66$, $p = 0.04$);
- Decrease in MDA in the OCC-COO group ($F = 3.74$, $p = 0.01$) and CONT group ($F = 3.12$, $p = 0.03$); T-AOC in the OCC-COO group ($F = 3.96$, $p = 0.01$), OCC group ($F = 7.24$, $p = 0.00$) and the CONT group ($F = 2.76$, $p = 0.04$); PT Quick in the OCC-

COO group (F = 17.45, p = 0.00), the OCC group (F = 8.27, p = 0.00) and CONT group (F = 6.51, p = 0.00); INR in the OCC-COO group (F = 3.28, p = 0.01), OCC group (F = 4.22, p = 0.00) and CONT group (F = 2.67, p = 0.05); and TT in the OCC-COO group (F = 4.31, p = 0.00).

Statistical analysis of changes in the average values of indicators in all study groups showed a significant change increase due to the time of testing IGF-1 (F = 2.37, p = 0.04), XOD (F = 14.26, p = 0.00), D-Dimer (F = 2.90, p = 0.02), and decrease in MDA (F = 7.14, p = 0.00), T-AOC (F = 11.17, p = 0.00), PT Quick (F = 26.37, p = 0.00), INR (F = 8.79, p = 0.00), TT (F = 3.81, p = 0.00).

Table 1. Tested indicators (mean ± standard deviation).

Parameters	Group	I	II	III	IV	V	VI
HGH [ng/mL]	OCC-COO	1.23 ± 0.79	6.64 ± 14.62	6.83 ± 10.51	1.18 ± 1.01	1.41 ± 1.27	1.21 ± 0.78
	OCC	3.64 ± 5.53	4.66 ± 9.64	3.45 ± 4.86	7.02 ± 12.90	2.05 ± 3.29	3.53 ± 7.93
	CONT	2.06 ± 1.25	1.27 ± 0.78	1.15 ± 0.88	1.42 ± 1.13	2.46 ± 2.70	2.04 ± 2.82
IGF-1 [ng/mL]	OCC-COO	84.27 ± 17.11	83.49 ± 20.48	88.97 ± 22.16	95.18 ± 49.15	147.50 ± 75.62	117.90 ± 43.82
	OCC	85.35 ± 11.71	96.27 ± 28.76	94.96 ± 37.09	116.05 ± 62.60	117.54 ± 42.13	131.81 ± 60.50
	CONT	120.76 ± 50.52	92.89 ± 39.38	105.85 ± 29.30	147.61 ± 49.20	99.78 ± 51.50	115.35 ± 65.21
MDA [nmol/mL]	OCC-COO	4.30 ± 1.81	4.06 ± 1.83	3.45 ± 2.27	2.75 ± 1.13	3.60 ± 1.92	2.73 ± 1.80
	OCC	3.84 ± 1.16	3.43 ± 1.56	3.32 ± 1.01	2.45 ± 1.04	3.26 ± 1.42	2.89 ± 1.24
	CONT	4.55 ± 1.86	3.57 ± 1.12	3.24 ± 0.95	3.44 ± 1.08	2.86 ± 1.85	2.85 ± 1.04
T-AOC [U/mL]	OCC-COO	6.91 ± 3.98	6.88 ± 2.25	7.57 ± 3.34	3.98 ± 1.88	4.00 ± 1.25	5.91 ± 3.17
	OCC	5.87 ± 3.48	7.61 ± 2.37	6.07 ± 2.90	3.61 ± 1.78	4.62 ± 2.76	3.15 ± 2.20
	CONT	6.14 ± 1.51	8.84 ± 5.60	7.35 ± 5.39	3.55 ± 1.33	4.67 ± 2.25	3.33 ± 1.61
TOS [U/mL]	OCC-COO	25.97 ± 9.03	30.07 ± 17.30	31.71 ± 13.43	25.96 ± 6.51	36.36 ± 20.72	37.56 ± 17.75
	OCC	24.38 ± 13.95	33.41 ± 18.83	39.92 ± 20.17	63.33 ± 101.49	68.12 ± 102.31	25.53 ± 6.66
	CONT	40.51 ± 14.44	31.35 ± 9.56	28.39 ± 11.78	31.97 ± 8.43	33.84 ± 5.00	81.06 ± 142.98
VEGF [ng/L]	OCC-COO	857.52 ± 258.86	837.71 ± 281.89	745.30 ± 285.13	953.71 ± 395.19	911.27 ± 424.97	834.30 ± 239.77
	OCC	891.03 ± 265.45	997.31 ± 349.36	744.82 ± 268.71	1183.08 ± 681.44	976.39 ± 442.41	900.97 ± 436.82
	CONT	753.57 ± 162.34	906.42 ± 380.74	830.65 ± 223.52	861.13 ± 280.11	800.30 ± 116.45	985.13 ± 375.70
XOD [ng/mL]	OCC-COO	17.18 ± 3.82	13.06 ± 3.53	14.16 ± 1.93	25.96 ± 10.02	21.21 ± 5.63	20.07 ± 3.50
	OCC	15.82 ± 3.08	16.50 ± 5.08	12.98 ± 1.86	21.94 ± 9.05	24.93 ± 11.62	21.79 ± 8.77
	CONT	16.23 ± 3.87	14.73 ± 4.19	13.76 ± 2.55	19.18 ± 4.87	24.22 ± 5.96	16.70 ± 4.61
CORT [µg/dL]	OCC-COO	18.10 ± 4.71	18.61 ± 2.40	16.32 ± 2.31	17.52 ± 1.79	17.63 ± 1.44	18.19 ± 1.65
	OCC	19.72 ± 4.19	19.04 ± 5.49	18.38 ± 2.30	18.09 ± 2.69	18.37 ± 2.81	17.57 ± 2.49
	CONT	19.42 ± 4.78	20.05 ± 3.21	18.08 ± 4.13	21.12 ± 2.98	20.75 ± 5.14	19.72 ± 4.10
MIO [µg/L]	OCC-COO	40.13 ± 29.22	31.79 ± 8.43	37.01 ± 18.04	34.76 ± 13.06	34.07 ± 14.92	32.71 ± 8.48
	OCC	40.99 ± 19.57	36.98 ± 14.65	37.22 ± 17.62	34.01 ± 13.41	28.53 ± 9.47	60.69 ± 86.90
	CONT	25.67 ± 6.12	29.63 ± 12.63	28.83 ± 12.27	36.40 ± 23.88	27.87 ± 5.72	33.45 ± 18.23
PT Quick [%]	OCC-COO	99.41 ± 9.63	100.87 ± 7.18	95.25 ± 8.20	90.96 ± 7.70	90.94 ± 8.83	89.03 ± 7.30
	OCC	104.45 ± 10.80	104.60 ± 14.94	99.58 ± 16.48	91.73 ± 16.70	95.70 ± 14.19	95.81 ± 16.20
	CONT	101.20 ± 8.82	101.37 ± 11.00	97.80 ± 6.09	90.38 ± 6.91	93.97 ± 8.59	91.58 ± 9.39
INR	OCC-COO	1.12 ± 0.07	1.08 ± 0.05	1.09 ± 0.05	1.12 ± 0.05	1.12 ± 0.06	1.10 ± 0.05
	OCC	1.09 ± 0.07	1.06 ± 0.08	1.07 ± 0.11	1.13 ± 0.12	1.10 ± 0.09	1.06 ± 0.08
	CONT	1.11 ± 0.06	1.08 ± 0.06	1.08 ± 0.04	1.13 ± 0.05	1.10 ± 0.06	1.08 ± 0.06

Table 1. Cont.

Parameters	Group	I	II	III	IV	V	VI
aPTT [s]	OCC-COO	29.40 ± 1.72	29.80 ± 1.80	29.88 ± 2.45	29.42 ± 1.32	29.87 ± 1.75	29.39 ± 1.77
	OCC	28.17 ± 2.87	28.50 ± 3.13	29.12 ± 3.68	28.73 ± 3.62	28.73 ± 4.00	28.42 ± 3.21
	CONT	27.98 ± 1.11	28.07 ± 1.89	28.53 ± 1.03	28.37 ± 0.70	27.65 ± 1.48	27.62 ± 1.69
Fibrinogen [g/L]	OCC-COO	2.32 ± 0.27	2.30 ± 0.51	2.15 ± 0.32	2.78 ± 0.83	2.39 ± 0.29	2.29 ± 0.20
	OCC	2.78 ± 0.66	2.55 ± 0.41	2.43 ± 0.27	2.44 ± 0.53	2.51 ± 0.69	2.71 ± 0.82
	CONT	2.76 ± 0.69	2.69 ± 0.84	2.57 ± 0.69	2.85 ± 0.95	2.77 ± 0.76	2.63 ± 0.68
D-Dimer [mg/L]	OCC-COO	0.20 ± 0.04	0.23 ± 0.08	0.28 ± 0.18	0.20 ± 0.06	0.38 ± 0.24	0.28 ± 0.21
	OCC	0.28 ± 0.17	0.28 ± 0.19	0.24 ± 0.13	0.24 ± 0.13	0.29 ± 0.20	0.25 ± 0.13
	CONT	0.27 ± 0.10	0.30 ± 0.14	0.27 ± 0.11	0.26 ± 0.11	0.34 ± 0.17	0.29 ± 0.18
TT [s]	OCC-COO	18.12 ± 0.79	18.39 ± 1.14	18.80 ± 0.86	17.22 ± 1.21	18.79 ± 0.77	18.07 ± 0.99
	OCC	17.62 ± 1.23	18.08 ± 1.21	18.20 ± 1.07	18.29 ± 1.44	18.50 ± 1.43	17.73 ± 1.07
	CONT	17.30 ± 1.39	17.77 ± 1.16	17.90 ± 0.88	17.45 ± 1.58	18.42 ± 1.21	17.85 ± 0.95

HGH (Human Growth Hormone), IGF-1 (Insulin-like Growth Factor 1), VEGF (Vascular Endothelial Growth Factor), MDA (Malondialdehyde), T-AOC (Total Antioxidant Capacity), TOS (Total Oxidative Status), XOD (Xanthine Oxidase), CORT (Cortisol), MIO (Myoglobin), PT Quick, INR (International Normalized Ratio), aPTT (Activated Partial Thromboplastin Time), TT (Thrombin Time).

Table 2. Analysis of variance for repeated measurements for the studied indicators in groups—F test value and significance level p.

Parameters	Groups	F Test Value	Significance Level p
HGH [ng/mL]	OCC-COO	1.58	0.19
	OCC	0.84	0.53
	CONT	0.65	0.66
IGF-1 [ng/mL]	OCC-COO	2.85	0.03
	OCC	1.44	0.23
	CONT	0.96	0.46
MDA [nmol/mL]	OCC-COO	3.74	0.01
	OCC	2.30	0.06
	CONT	3.12	0.03
T-AOC [U/mL]	OCC-COO	3.96	0.01
	OCC	7.24	0.00
	CONT	2.76	0.04
TOS [U/mL]	OCC-COO	1.30	0.28
	OCC	1.11	0.37
	CONT	0.70	0.63
VEGF [ng/L]	OCC-COO	0.57	0.72
	OCC	1.17	0.34
	CONT	0.78	0.57
XOD [ng/mL]	OCC-COO	10.69	0.00
	OCC	4.42	0.00
	CONT	6.48	0.00
CORT [µg/dL]	OCC-COO	0.94	0.46
	OCC	0.94	0.46
	CONT	2.11	0.10

Table 2. Cont.

Parameters	Groups	F Test Value	Significance Level p
MIO [μg/L]	OCC-COO	0.40	0.84
	OCC	0.85	0.53
	CONT	1.03	0.42
PT Quick [%]	OCC-COO	17.45	0.00
	OCC	8.27	0.00
	CONT	6.51	0.00
INR	OCC-COO	3.28	0.01
	OCC	4.22	0.00
	CONT	2.67	0.05
aPTT [s]	OCC-COO	0.59	0.71
	OCC	1.36	0.26
	CONT	0.85	0.53
Fibrinogen [g/L]	OCC-COO	2.81	0.03
	OCC	0.97	0.45
	CONT	0.41	0.84
D-Dimer [mg/L]	OCC-COO	2.66	0.04
	OCC	0.57	0.72
	CONT	1.26	0.31
TT [s]	OCC-COO	4.31	0.00
	OCC	1.77	0.14
	CONT	0.73	0.61

HGH (Human Growth Hormone), IGF-1 (Insulin-like Growth Factor 1), VEGF (Vascular Endothelial Growth Factor), MDA (Malondialdehyde), T-AOC (Total Antioxidant Capacity), TOS (Total Oxidative Status), XOD (Xanthine Oxidase), CORT (Cortisol), MIO (Myoglobin), PT Quick, INR (International Normalized Ratio), aPTT (Activated Partial Thromboplastin Time), TT (Thrombin Time). ANOVA test for repeated measurements was performed; significance level of $p = 0.05$.

Table 3. Post hoc test values for the studied indicators depending on the study in the same groups.

Parameters	Study	I	II	III	IV	V	VI
IGF-1 [ng/mL] OCC-COO	I		0.97	0.83	0.61	0.00	0.12
	II	0.97		0.80	0.58	0.00	0.11
	III	0.83	0.80		0.77	0.01	0.18
	IV	0.61	0.58	0.77		0.02	0.29
	V	0.00	0.00	0.01	0.02		0.17
	VI	0.12	0.11	0.18	0.29	0.17	
MDA [nmol/mL] OCC-COO	I		0.62	0.08	0.00	0.15	0.00
	II	0.62		0.21	0.01	0.33	0.01
	III	0.08	0.21		0.15	0.76	0.14
	IV	0.00	0.01	0.15		0.08	0.98
	V	0.15	0.33	0.76	0.08		0.08
	VI	0.00	0.01	0.14	0.98	0.08	

Table 3. Cont.

Parameters	Study	I	II	III	IV	V	VI
MDA [nmol/mL] CONT	I		0.06	0.02	0.04	0.00	0.00
	II	0.06		0.51	0.79	0.17	0.16
	III	0.02	0.51		0.69	0.46	0.44
	IV	0.04	0.79	0.69		0.26	0.25
	V	0.00	0.17	0.46	0.26		0.98
	VI	0.00	0.16	0.44	0.25	0.98	
T-AOC [U/mL] OCC-COO	I		0.98	0.55	0.01	0.01	0.37
	II	0.98		0.53	0.01	0.01	0.38
	III	0.55	0.53		0.00	0.00	0.14
	IV	0.01	0.01	0.00		0.99	0.09
	V	0.01	0.01	0.00	0.99		0.09
	VI	0.37	0.38	0.14	0.09	0.09	
T-AOC [U/mL] OCC	I		0.06	0.83	0.01	0.16	0.00
	II	0.06		0.09	0.00	0.00	0.00
	III	0.83	0.09		0.01	0.11	0.00
	IV	0.01	0.00	0.01		0.26	0.61
	V	0.16	0.00	0.11	0.26		0.10
	VI	0.00	0.00	0.00	0.61	0.10	
T-AOC [U/mL] CONT	I		0.16	0.52	0.18	0.44	0.14
	II	0.16		0.43	0.01	0.04	0.01
	III	0.52	0.43		0.05	0.16	0.04
	IV	0.18	0.01	0.05		0.55	0.90
	V	0.44	0.04	0.16	0.55		0.48
	VI	0.14	0.01	0.04	0.90	0.48	
XOD [ng/mL] OCC-COO	I		0.05	0.15	0.00	0.06	0.17
	II	0.05		0.60	0.00	0.00	0.00
	III	0.15	0.60		0.00	0.00	0.01
	IV	0.00	0.00	0.00		0.03	0.01
	V	0.06	0.00	0.00	0.03		0.59
	VI	0.17	0.00	0.01	0.01	0.59	
XOD [ng/mL] OCC	I		0.83	0.36	0.05	0.01	0.06
	II	0.83		0.26	0.08	0.01	0.09
	III	0.36	0.26		0.01	0.00	0.01
	IV	0.05	0.08	0.01		0.34	0.96
	V	0.01	0.01	0.00	0.34		0.31
	VI	0.06	0.09	0.01	0.96	0.31	
XOD [ng/mL] CONT	I		0.48	0.25	0.17	0.00	0.82
	II	0.48		0.65	0.05	0.00	0.36
	III	0.25	0.65		0.02	0.00	0.17
	IV	0.17	0.05	0.02		0.02	0.25
	V	0.00	0.00	0.00	0.02		0.00
	VI	0.82	0.36	0.17	0.25	0.00	

Table 3. Cont.

Parameters	Study	I	II	III	IV	V	VI
PT Quick [%] OCC-COO	I		0.38	0.02	0.00	0.00	0.00
	II	0.38		0.00	0.00	0.00	0.00
	III	0.02	0.00		0.01	0.01	0.00
	IV	0.00	0.00	0.01		0.99	0.25
	V	0.00	0.00	0.01	0.99		0.26
	VI	0.00	0.00	0.00	0.25	0.26	
PT Quick [%] OCC	I		0.95	0.06	0.00	0.00	0.00
	II	0.95		0.06	0.00	0.00	0.00
	III	0.06	0.06		0.00	0.14	0.15
	IV	0.00	0.00	0.00		0.13	0.12
	V	0.00	0.00	0.14	0.13		0.96
	VI	0.00	0.00	0.15	0.12	0.96	
PT Quick [%] CONT	I		0.95	0.21	0.00	0.01	0.00
	II	0.95		0.19	0.00	0.01	0.00
	III	0.21	0.19		0.01	0.16	0.03
	IV	0.00	0.00	0.01		0.19	0.65
	V	0.01	0.01	0.16	0.19		0.38
	VI	0.00	0.00	0.03	0.65	0.38	
INR OCC-COO	I		0.01	0.06	1.00	1.00	0.08
	II	0.01		0.32	0.01	0.01	0.25
	III	0.06	0.32		0.06	0.06	0.88
	IV	1.00	0.01	0.06		1.00	0.08
	V	1.00	0.01	0.06	1.00		0.08
	VI	0.08	0.25	0.88	0.08	0.08	
INR OCC	I		0.11	0.42	0.04	0.66	0.11
	II	0.11		0.42	0.00	0.04	1.00
	III	0.42	0.42		0.00	0.21	0.42
	IV	0.04	0.00	0.00		0.10	0.00
	V	0.66	0.04	0.21	0.10		0.04
	VI	0.11	1.00	0.42	0.00	0.04	
INR CONT	I		0.09	0.06	0.34	0.70	0.13
	II	0.09		0.85	0.01	0.19	0.85
	III	0.06	0.85		0.01	0.13	0.70
	IV	0.34	0.01	0.01		0.19	0.02
	V	0.70	0.19	0.13	0.19		0.26
	VI	0.13	0.85	0.70	0.02	0.26	
Fibrinogen [g/L] OCC-COO	I		0.94	0.36	0.01	0.69	0.88
	II	0.94		0.40	0.01	0.64	0.94
	III	0.36	0.40		0.00	0.19	0.45
	IV	0.01	0.01	0.00		0.04	0.01
	V	0.69	0.64	0.19	0.04		0.58
	VI	0.88	0.94	0.45	0.01	0.58	

Table 3. Cont.

Parameters	Study	I	II	III	IV	V	VI
D-Dimer [mg/L] OCC-COO	I		0.60	0.18	0.99	0.00	0.19
	II	0.60		0.40	0.59	0.02	0.43
	III	0.18	0.40		0.17	0.10	0.97
	IV	0.99	0.59	0.17		0.00	0.18
	V	0.00	0.02	0.10	0.00		0.10
	VI	0.19	0.43	0.97	0.18	0.10	
TT [s] OCC-COO	I		0.51	0.10	0.03	0.10	0.89
	II	0.51		0.31	0.01	0.32	0.42
	III	0.10	0.31		0.00	0.98	0.07
	IV	0.03	0.01	0.00		0.00	0.04
	V	0.10	0.32	0.98	0.00		0.08
	VI	0.89	0.42	0.07	0.04	0.08	

IGF-1 (Insulin-like Growth Factor 1), MDA (Malondialdehyde), T-AOC (Total Antioxidant Capacity), XOD (Xanthine Oxidase), PT Quick, INR (International Normalized Ratio), TT (Thrombin Time). NIR post hoc test was performed; significance level of $p = 0.05$.

Table 4. Multivariate analysis of variance for repeated measurements for the studied indicators between groups—F test value and significance level p depending on the factor used.

Parameters	Factor	F Test Value	Significance Level p
HGH [ng/mL]	S	0.66	0.66
	I	0.45	0.65
	S*I	1.20	0.30
IGF-1 [ng/mL]	S	2.37	0.04
	I	0.69	0.51
	S*I	1.22	0.29
MDA [nmol/mL]	S	7.14	0.00
	I	0.12	0.88
	S*I	0.81	0.62
T-AOC [U/mL]	S	11.17	0.00
	I	0.34	0.72
	S*I	1.01	0.44
TOS [U/mL]	S	0.69	0.63
	I	0.50	0.62
	S*I	1.14	0.34
VEGF [ng/L]	S	1.30	0.27
	I	0.59	0.57
	S*I	0.53	0.87
XOD [ng/mL]	S	14.26	0.00
	I	0.29	0.75
	S*I	1.32	0.23

Table 4. *Cont.*

Parameters	Factor	F Test Value	Significance Level *p*
CORT [µg/dL]	S	1.60	0.17
	I	1.15	0.34
	S*I	0.94	0.50
MIO [µg/L]	S	0.64	0.67
	I	0.75	0.48
	S*I	0.69	0.73
PT Quick [%]	S	26.37	0.00
	I	0.37	0.70
	S*I	0.49	0.89
INR	S	8.79	0.00
	I	0.29	0.75
	S*I	0.54	0.86
aPTT [s]	S	1.75	0.13
	I	0.90	0.42
	S*I	0.48	0.90
Fibrinogen [g/L]	S	1.51	0.19
	I	1.00	0.38
	S*I	1.20	0.30
D-Dimer [mg/L]	S	2.90	0.02
	I	0.09	0.91
	S*I	1.06	0.40
TT [s]	S	3.81	0.00
	I	0.56	0.58
	S*I	1.20	0.30

HGH (Human Growth Hormone), IGF-1 (Insulin-like Growth Factor 1), VEGF (Vascular Endothelial Growth Factor), MDA (Malondialdehyde), T-AOC (Total Antioxidant Capacity), TOS (Total Oxidative Status), XOD (Xanthine Oxidase), CORT (Cortisol), MIO (Myoglobin), PT Quick, INR (International Normalized Ratio), aPTT (Activated Partial Thromboplastin Time), TT (Thrombin Time), S-Study, I-Intervention, S*I—Study*Intervention. Multivariate ANOVA test was performed; significance level of $p = 0.05$.

Table 5. Post hoc test values for the studied indicators depending on the study between groups.

Parameters	Study	I	II	III	IV	V	VI
IGF-1 [ng/mL]	I		0.81	0.90	0.09	0.02	0.03
	II	0.81		0.71	0.05	0.01	0.02
	III	0.90	0.71		0.12	0.03	0.04
	IV	0.09	0.05	0.12		0.53	0.63
	V	0.02	0.01	0.03	0.53		0.89
	VI	0.03	0.02	0.04	0.63	0.89	
MDA [nmol/mL]	I		0.08	0.00	0.00	0.00	0.00
	II	0.08		0.20	0.00	0.13	0.00
	III	0.00	0.20		0.05	0.82	0.06
	IV	0.00	0.00	0.05		0.09	0.97

Table 5. *Cont.*

Parameters	Study	I	II	III	IV	V	VI
MDA [nmol/mL]	V	0.00	0.13	0.82	0.09		0.09
	VI	0.00	0.00	0.06	0.97	0.09	
T-AOC [U/mL]	I		0.06	0.37	0.00	0.01	0.00
	II	0.06		0.33	0.00	0.00	0.00
	III	0.37	0.33		0.00	0.00	0.00
	IV	0.00	0.00	0.00		0.35	0.48
	V	0.01	0.00	0.00	0.35		0.81
	VI	0.00	0.00	0.00	0.48	0.81	
XOD [ng/mL]	I		0.27	0.06	0.00	0.00	0.02
	II	0.27		0.44	0.00	0.00	0.00
	III	0.06	0.44		0.00	0.00	0.00
	IV	0.00	0.00	0.00		0.69	0.06
	V	0.00	0.00	0.00	0.69		0.02
	VI	0.02	0.00	0.00	0.06	0.02	
PT Quick [%]	I		0.62	0.00	0.00	0.00	0.00
	II	0.62		0.00	0.00	0.00	0.00
	III	0.00	0.00		0.00	0.00	0.00
	IV	0.00	0.00	0.00		0.07	0.40
	V	0.00	0.00	0.00	0.07		0.34
	VI	0.00	0.00	0.00	0.40	0.34	
INR	I		0.00	0.01	0.06	0.90	0.01
	II	0.00		0.30	0.00	0.00	0.46
	III	0.01	0.30		0.00	0.01	0.76
	IV	0.06	0.00	0.00		0.08	0.00
	V	0.90	0.00	0.01	0.08		0.00
	VI	0.01	0.46	0.76	0.00	0.00	
D-Dimer [mg/L]	I		0.50	0.56	0.53	0.00	0.42
	II	0.50		0.93	0.20	0.02	0.88
	III	0.56	0.93		0.23	0.01	0.82
	IV	0.53	0.20	0.23		0.00	0.15
	V	0.00	0.02	0.01	0.00		0.03
	VI	0.42	0.88	0.82	0.15	0.03	
TT [s]	I		0.13	0.02	0.85	0.00	0.54
	II	0.13		0.37	0.09	0.07	0.37
	III	0.02	0.37		0.01	0.36	0.07
	IV	0.85	0.09	0.01		0.00	0.42
	V	0.00	0.07	0.36	0.00		0.01
	VI	0.54	0.37	0.07	0.42	0.01	

IGF-1 (Insulin-like Growth Factor 1), MDA (Malondialdehyde), T-AOC (Total Antioxidant Capacity), XOD (Xanthine Oxidase), PT Quick, INR (International Normalized Ratio), TT (Thrombin Time). NIR post hoc test was performed; significance level of $p = 0.05$.

4. Discussion

Physical exercise, mainly aerobic, is a well-researched method of strengthening the capillary network in skeletal muscles [23]. There is also evidence that high-intensity resistance exercise also induces angiogenic signaling in activated muscles [24]. An increase in VEGF levels, which is considered an important modulator of vasculogenesis and angiogenesis, is necessary for hypertrophy and can be stimulated by lactate accumulation and hypoxia [25–28]. There is also evidence of an increase in the rate of angiogenesis when lactate levels are increased, thus producing an even greater hypertrophic stimulus [29]. Accordingly, lactate accumulation resulting from occlusion-induced hypoxia is a stimulus for muscle hypertrophy. Larkin et al. (2012) assessed the post-exercise VEGF level in serum during unilateral knee extension with and without the addition of BFR. They also examined mRNA transcripts indicating angiogenesis, i.e.,: VEGF and its main receptor (VEGF-R2), hypoxia-inducible factor 1 alpha (HIF-1alpha) and nitric oxide synthase isoforms (NOS) [30]. The key finding was that the BFR condition induced a significantly greater angiogenic response compared with the non-BFR condition. Although serum VEGF levels did not differ significantly between groups, mRNA transcripts for VEGF, VEGF-R2, and neuronal nitric oxide synthase were significantly greater at BFR at 4 and 24 h postexercise. In our studies, we observed trends towards lower VEGF 24 h after the first training, and higher concentrations only after the 10th and 20th training, but these changes were not statistically significant.

Muscle hypertrophy and increased strength after a single high-intensity exercise session are thought to be related to the recruitment of high-threshold motor units [31,32]. The recruitment of these motor units results in a significant increase in mechanical stress [33,34] and endocrine responses [35], as well as the accumulation of metabolites [36]. It is hypothesized that the accumulation of metabolic byproducts and/or the hypoxia-induced stimulation of afferent nerve fibers causes an increase in the secretion of GH and GH-releasing hormone [37]. Kraemer and Ratamess (2005) found that a large, sharp increase in GH after exercise stimulates IGF secretion, leading to increased protein synthesis and ultimately muscle hypertrophy [38]. Pierce et al. (2006) observed a nine-fold increase in serum GH concentration from baseline to the cessation of knee extension exercises using BFR [39]. There are also studies that report increases in GH up to 290 times the baseline [14,40–42], with the GH response after BFR and low-intensity exercise being similar or even higher than that observed during high-intensity exercise [38,43]. It has been suggested that lactate accumulation plays a key role in GH release during exercise, which is supported by the fact that people lacking the myophosphorylase enzyme (those who do not show an increase in blood lactate levels during exercise) show a weaker GH response [44]. However, Reeves et al. (2006) demonstrated an increased GH response in the BFR training group compared to traditional non-BFR training groups with the same lactate concentrations [45], suggesting additional mechanisms. IGF-1 production also increases with GH. In fact, IGF-1 increases protein synthesis and activates satellite cells, which causes myofibril hypertrophy [46]. Furthermore, muscle hypertrophy occurred with the viral overexpression of IGF-1 [47]. The increase in IGF1 observed in some studies may be related to hemoconcentration due to changes in plasma volume after BFR resistance exercise [48]. After a training series, a progressive increase in IGF1 levels was observed after 2 weeks of twice-daily BFR exercise [49]. Therefore, the overall relationship between BFR resistance exercise and the GH–IGF1 axis remains controversial. West et al. (2009) reported no increase in muscle protein synthesis or the phosphorylation of signaling proteins after resistance exercise with elevated systemic concentrations of T, GH, and IGF1 compared to low systemic concentrations of the same anabolic hormones [50]. An important mechanism underlying BFR-induced hypertrophy may be the prolonged duration of metabolic acidosis, which induces systemic GH release. Abe et al. (2005) reported an increased IGF-1 response to low-intensity resistance training with BFR. The control group in this study performed a protocol of the same intensity and volume but did not show a similar response [49]. In our studies, we observed a statistically significant increase in IGF-1 after completed training in the occlusion and cooling group; in the occlusion-only group, an increasing tendency was also observed, although statistically insignificant. When analyzing HGH, we did not note any statistically significant changes.

The stress of resistance exercise is known to increase cortisol levels. Fujita et al. (2007) compared four sets of exercises with and without BFR. The authors found increased cortisol concentration after the BFR protocol compared to the control session. In this study, higher cortisol levels after the BFR session likely indicated a stronger stress response; this is evident by the fact that cortisol levels returned to baseline values approximately 1 h after exercise [51]. In our study, we did not observe changes in CORT over time or differences between groups.

The effects of resistance exercise combined with occlusion on systemic physiological markers of muscle damage are not well understood. Although no increased levels of creatine kinase and myoglobin were observed after two sets of resistance exercises with BFR [14,51], there are studies that report rhabdomyolysis [52]. In addition to the potential for muscle damage during BFR training, there is a hypothetical risk of microvascular dysfunction due to reperfusion, which occurs when blood flow is restored after a period of stenosis or ischemia [53]. It is hypothesized that during occlusion, a hypoxic and ischemic muscle environment is created, which causes high levels of metabolic stress as well as mechanical stress when BFR is used in conjunction with exercise. Both metabolic stress and mechanical stress have been described as "major factors of hypertrophy" [54] and have been assumed to activate other mechanisms to induce muscle growth: cell swelling [55], increased systemic hormone production [6,45], the production of reactive oxygen species (ROS) [51,56], the increased recruitment of fast-twitch fibers [57,58] and the intramuscular transmission of anabolic/anti-catabolic signals [18,41,59]. Additionally, although not statistically significant, Goldfarb et al. (2008) showed that the ratio of protein carbonyls and glutathione (systemic indicators of oxidative stress) increased almost twofold after BFR resistance exercise in a small group of men [60]. Analyzing the oxidative stress indicators in our subjects, we observed a decrease in MDA, statistically significant only in the CONT group, an increase in XOD in all groups after 10 and 20 training sessions and a decrease in T-AOC in all groups after 10 and 20 training sessions without a simultaneous change in TOS.

To the best of our knowledge, this study is the first to evaluate the effects of interval training combined with occlusion or occlusion and cooling on indices of muscle metabolism and oxidative stress in young healthy humans.

Study Limitation: The current experiment was not without flaws related to the lack of a uniform diet and its monitoring (the inclusion criterion was only the lack of change in diet before and during the project), but it undoubtedly showed the impact of interval training and its modifications on the tested indicators. Research should continue in groups of patients divided by gender and be adapted for people with vascular diseases and athletes.

5. Conclusions

Based on the research conducted, the following conclusions can be drawn:

- Changes in the examined indicators (IGF-1, MDA, T-AOC, XOD, PT Quick, INR, Fibrinogen, D-Dimer, and TT) were observed after a series of training sessions, not after a single training unit.
- Both interval training without and with the modifications used in the study influence coagulation (PT Quick, INR, Fibrinogen, D-Dimer, and TT) and oxidative stress (MDA, T-AOC, and XOD) parameters and, to a small extent, muscle metabolism (IGF-1).
- It seems reasonable to use occlusion and local cryotherapy in combination with occlusion.

Author Contributions: Conceptualization, B.P., S.P., O.C.-L., B.Z., R.N., P.M. and A.T.; methodology, B.P., S.P. and O.C.-L.; formal analysis, B.P. and S.P.; investigation, B.P. and S.P.; data curation, B.P., S.P. and O.C.-L.; writing—original draft preparation, B.P. and S.P.; writing—review and editing, B.P.;

supervision, P.M.; project administration, B.P. and S.P.; funding acquisition, B.P. and S.P. All authors have read and agreed to the published version of the manuscript.

Funding: The project is financed within the program of the Minister of Science and Higher Education in Poland under the name "Regional Excellence Initiative" in the years 2019–2022 (project number: 022/RID/2018/19) in the amount of PLN 11,919,908.

Institutional Review Board Statement: To conduct the research experiment, consent was obtained from the Bioethics Committee at the Regional Medical Chamber in Krakow—consent number: 164/KBL/OIL/2021. The trials were also registered with the ANZCTR (Australian New Zealand Clinical Trials Registry): ACTRN12622000734763.

Informed Consent Statement: Informed consent was obtained from all subjects involved in the study.

Data Availability Statement: All data generated or analyzed during this study are included in this published article.

Acknowledgments: Thanks to the company for lending the device for testing: BGP Sp. z o.o., Rynek 16/2, 35-064 Rzeszów.

Conflicts of Interest: The authors declare no conflict of interest.

References

1. Jawień, A.; Grzela, T.; Ciecierski, M.; Piotrowicz, R.; Szotkiewicz, A.; Migdalski, A. Buflomedil associated with pentoxiflylline in the treatment of patients with intermittent claudication. Opened, randomised, one-center-based study. *Acta Angiol.* 2003, *3*, 109–122.
2. Conte, M.S.; Bradbury, A.W.; Kolh, P.; White, J.V.; Dick, F.; Fitridge, R.; Mills, J.L.; Ricco, J.B.; Suresh, K.R.; Murad, M.H.; et al. Global vascular guidelines on the management of chronic limb-threatening ischemia. *J. Vasc. Surg.* 2019, *58*, S1–S109.
3. Frank, U.; Nikol, S.; Belch, J.; Boc, V.; Brodmann, M.; Carpentier, P.H.; Chraim, A.; Canning, C.; Dimakakos, E.; Gottsäter, A.; et al. ESVM Guideline on peripheral arterial disease. *Vasa* 2019, *48*, 1–79. [CrossRef] [PubMed]
4. Manini, T.M.; Clark, B.C. Blood Flow Restricted Exercise and Skeletal Muscle Health. *Exerc. Sport Sci. Rev.* 2009, *37*, 78–85. [CrossRef] [PubMed]
5. Hylden, C.; Burns, T.; Stinner, D.J.; Owens, J. Blood flow restriction rehabilitation for extremity weakness: A case series. *J. Spec. Oper. Med.* 2015, *15*, 50–56. [CrossRef] [PubMed]
6. Loenneke, J.; Fahs, C.; Rossow, L.; Abe, T.; Bemben, M. The anabolic benefits of venous blood flow restriction training may be induced by muscle cell swelling. *Med. Hypothes.* 2012, *78*, 151–154. [CrossRef]
7. Loenneke, J.; Fahs, C.; Wilson, J.; Bemben, M. Blood flow restriction: The metabolite/volume threshold theory. *Med. Hypothes.* 2011, *77*, 748–752. [CrossRef]
8. Loenneke, J.P.; Pujol, T.J. The Use of Occlusion Training to Produce Muscle Hypertrophy. *Strength Cond. J.* 2009, *31*, 77–84. [CrossRef]
9. Yasuda, T.; Fukumura, K.; Fukuda, T.; Iida, H.; Imuta, H.; Sato, Y.; Yamasoba, T.; Nakajima, T. Effects of low-intensity, elastic band resistance exercise combined with blood flow restriction on muscle activation. *Scand. J. Med. Sci. Sports* 2014, *24*, 55–61. [CrossRef]
10. Kang, D.Y.; Kim, H.S.; Lee, K.S.; Kim, Y.M. The effects of bodyweight-based exercise with blood flow restriction on isokinetic knee muscular function and thigh circumference in college students. *J. Phys. Ther. Sci.* 2015, *27*, 2709–2712. [CrossRef]
11. Hackney, K.J.; Everett, M.; Scott, J.M.; Ploutz-Snyder, L. Blood flow-restricted exercise in space. *Extreme Physiol. Med.* 2012, *1*, 12. [CrossRef]
12. Patterson, S.D.; Leggate, M.; Nimmo, M.A.; Ferguson, R.A. Circulating hormone and cytokine response to low-load resistance training with blood flow restriction in older men. *Eur. J. Appl. Physiol.* 2013, *113*, 713–719. [CrossRef] [PubMed]
13. Tanimoto, M.; Madarame, H.; Ishii, N. Muscle oxygenation and plasma growth hormone concentration during and after resistance exercise: Comparison between "KAATSU" and other types of regimen. *Int. J. KAATSU Train. Res.* 2005, *1*, 51–56. [CrossRef]
14. Takarada, Y.; Nakamura, Y.; Aruga, S.; Onda, T.; Miyazaki, S.; Ishii, N.; D'souza, R.F.; Woodhead, J.S.T.; Zeng, N.; Blenkiron, C.; et al. Rapid increase in plasma growth hormone after low-intensity resistance exercise with vascular occlusion. *J. Appl. Physiol.* 2000, *88*, 61–65. [CrossRef] [PubMed]
15. Sato, Y.; Yoshitomi, A.; Abe, T. Acute growth hormone response to low-intensity KAATSU resistance exercise: Comparison between arm and leg. *Int. J. KAATSU Train. Res.* 2005, *1*, 45–50. [CrossRef]
16. Victor, R.G.; Seals, D.R.; Kaur, J.; Senador, D.; Krishnan, A.C.; Hanna, H.W.; Alvarez, A.; Machado, T.M.; O'Leary, D.S.; Altamimi, Y.H.; et al. Reflex stimulation of sympathetic outflow during rhythmic exercise in humans. *Am. J. Physiol. Circ. Physiol.* 1989, *257*, H2017–H2024. [CrossRef]
17. Gosselink, K.L.; Zhong, H.; Bigbee, A.J.; Grossman, E.J.; Pierce, J.R.; Clark, B.C.; Ploutz-Snyder, L.L.; Kanaley, J.A.; Arnaud, S.; Nemet, D.; et al. Skeletal muscle afferent regulation of bioassayable growth hormone in the rat pituitary. *J. Appl. Physiol.* 1998, *84*, 1425–1430. [CrossRef]

18. Fry, C.S.; Glynn, E.L.; Drummond, M.J.; Timmerman, K.L.; Fujita, S.; Abe, T.; Dhanani, S.; Volpi, E.; Rasmussen, B.B.; Pignanelli, C.; et al. Blood flow restriction exercise stimulates mTORC1 signaling and muscle protein synthesis in older men. *J. Appl. Physiol.* **2010**, *108*, 1199–1209. [CrossRef]
19. Lacka, K.; Czyzyk, A. Hormony a układ sercowo-naczyniowy [Hormones and the cardiovascular system]. *Endokrynol. Pol.* **2008**, *59*, 420–432.
20. Patterson, S.D.; Ferguson, R.A. Increase in calf post-occlusive blood flow and strength following short-term resistance exercise training with blood flow restriction in young women. *Eur. J. Appl. Physiol.* **2010**, *108*, 1025–1033. [CrossRef]
21. Marino, F.E. Methods, advantages, and limitations of body cooling for exercise performance. *Br. J. Sports Med.* **2002**, *36*, 89–94. [CrossRef]
22. Arngrímsson, S.Á.; Petitt, D.S.; Stueck, M.G.; Jorgensen, D.K.; Cureton, K.J. Cooling vest worn during active warm-up improves 5-km run performance in the heat. *J. Appl. Physiol.* **2004**, *96*, 1867–1874. [CrossRef]
23. Prior, B.M.; Lloyd, P.G.; Yang, H.T.; Terjung, R.L. Exercise-Induced Vascular Remodeling. *Exerc. Sport Sci. Rev.* **2003**, *31*, 26–33. [CrossRef] [PubMed]
24. Gavin, T.P.; Drew, J.L.; Kubik, C.J.; Pofahl, W.E.; Hickner, R.C. Acute resistance exercise increases skeletal muscle angiogenic growth factor expression. *Acta Physiol.* **2007**, *191*, 139–146. [CrossRef] [PubMed]
25. Drummond, M.J.; Fujita, S.; Takashi, A.; Dreyer, H.C.; Volpi, E.; Rasmussen, B.B. Human muscle gene expression following resistance exercise and blood flow restriction. *Med. Sci. Sports Exerc.* **2008**, *40*, 691–698. [CrossRef]
26. Gerber, H.-P.; Hillan, K.J.; Ryan, A.M.; Kowalski, J.; Keller, G.-A.; Rangell, L.; Wright, B.D.; Radtke, F.; Aguet, M.; Ferrara, N. VEGF is required for growth and survival in neonatal mice. *Development* **1999**, *126*, 1149–1159. [CrossRef] [PubMed]
27. Gerber, H.-P.; Vu, T.H.; Ryan, A.M.; Kowalski, J.; Werb, Z.; Ferrara, N. VEGF couples hypertrophic cartilage remodeling, ossification and angiogenesis during endochondral bone formation. *Nat. Med.* **1999**, *5*, 623–628. [CrossRef] [PubMed]
28. Semsarian, C.; Sutrave, P.; Richmond, D.R.; Graham, R.M. Insulin-like growth factor (IGF-I) induces myotube hypertrophy associated with an increase in anaerobic glycolysis in a clonal skeletal-muscle cell model. *Biochem. J.* **1999**, *339*, 443–451. [CrossRef] [PubMed]
29. Hunt, T.K.; Aslam, R.; Hussain, Z.; Beckert, S. Lactate, with oxygen, incites angiogenesis. *Adv. Exp. Med. Biol.* **2008**, *614*, 73–80. [PubMed]
30. Larkin, K.A.; Macneil, R.G.; Dirain, M.; Sandesara, B.; Manini, T.M.; Buford, T.W. Blood flow restriction enhances post–resistance exercise angiogenic gene expression. *Med. Sci. Sports Exerc.* **2012**, *44*, 2077–2083. [CrossRef]
31. Mackintosh, S.F.H.; Goldie, P.; Hill, K. Falls incidence and factors associated with falling in older, community-dwelling, chronic stroke survivors (>1 year after stroke) and matched controls. *Aging Clin. Exp. Res.* **2005**, *17*, 74–81. [CrossRef]
32. Mackintosh, S.F.; Hill, K.; Dodd, K.J.; Goldie, P.; Culham, E. Falls and injury prevention should be part of every stroke rehabilitation plan. *Clin. Rehabil.* **2005**, *19*, 441–451. [CrossRef]
33. Häkkinen, K. Neuromuscular fatigue and recovery in male and female athletes during heavy resistance exercise. *Int. J. Sports Med.* **1993**, *14*, 53–59. [CrossRef] [PubMed]
34. Häkkinen, K.; Pakarinen, A.; Suga, T.; Okita, K.; Morita, N.; Yokota, T.; Hirabayashi, K.; Horiuchi, M.; Takada, S.; Omokawa, M.; et al. Acute hormonal responses to two different fatiguing heavy-resistance protocols in male athletes. *J. Appl. Physiol.* **1993**, *74*, 882–887. [CrossRef]
35. Kraemer, R.R.; Hollander, D.B.; Reeves, G.V.; Francois, M.; Ramadan, Z.G.; Meeker, B.; Tryniecki, J.L.; Hebert, E.P.; Castracane, V.D. Similar hormonal responses to concentric and eccentric muscle actions using relative loading. *Eur. J. Appl. Physiol.* **2006**, *96*, 551–557. [CrossRef] [PubMed]
36. Jones, D.A.; Rutherford, O.M. Human muscle strength training: The effects of three different regimens and the nature of the resultant changes. *J. Physiol.* **1987**, *391*, 1–11. [CrossRef] [PubMed]
37. Takano, H.; Morita, T.; Iida, H.; Asada, K.-I.; Kato, M.; Uno, K.; Hirose, K.; Matsumoto, A.; Takenaka, K.; Hirata, Y.; et al. Hemodynamic and hormonal responses to a short-term low-intensity resistance exercise with the reduction of muscle blood flow. *Eur. J. Appl. Physiol.* **2005**, *95*, 65–73. [CrossRef]
38. Kraemer, W.J.; Ratamess, N.A. Hormonal Responses and Adaptations to Resistance Exercise and Training. *Sports Med.* **2005**, *35*, 339–361. [CrossRef]
39. Pierce, J.D.; Hall, S.; Clancy, R.L.; Goodyear-Bruch, C. Effect of dopamine on rat diaphragm apoptosis and muscle performance. *Exp. Physiol.* **2006**, *91*, 731–740. [CrossRef]
40. Takarada, Y.; Takazawa, H.; Sato, Y.; Takebayashi, S.; Tanaka, Y.; Ishii, N.; Mitchell, E.A.; Martin, N.R.W.; Turner, M.C.; Taylor, C.W.; et al. Effects of resistance exercise combined with moderate vascular occlusion on muscular function in humans. *J. Appl. Physiol.* **2000**, *88*, 2097–2106. [CrossRef]
41. Takarada, Y.; Sato, Y.; Ishii, N. Effects of resistance exercise combined with vascular occlusion on muscle function in athletes. *Eur. J. Appl. Physiol.* **2002**, *86*, 308–314. [CrossRef]
42. Takarada, Y.; Takazawa, H.; Ishii, N. Applications of vascular occlusion diminish disuse atrophy of knee extensor muscles. *Med. Sci. Sports Exerc.* **2000**, *32*, 2035–2039. [CrossRef]
43. Ploutz, L.L.; Tesch, P.A.; Biro, R.L.; Barrett-O'Keefe, Z.; Helgerud, J.; Wagner, P.D.; Richardson, R.S.; Giesebrecht, S.; van Duinen, H.; Todd, G.; et al. Effect of resistance training on muscle use during exercise. *J. Appl. Physiol.* **1994**, *76*, 1675–1681. [CrossRef]

44. Godfrey, R.J.; Whyte, G.P.; Buckley, J.; Quinlivan, R. The role of lactate in the exercise-induced human growth hormone response: Evidence from McArdle disease. *Br. J. Sports Med.* **2009**, *43*, 521–525. [CrossRef] [PubMed]
45. Reeves, G.V.; Kraemer, R.R.; Hollander, D.B.; Clavier, J.; Thomas, C.; Francois, M.; Castracane, V.D. Comparison of hormone responses following light resistance exercise with partial vascular occlusion and moderately difficult resistance exercise without occlusion. *J. Appl. Physiol.* **2006**, *101*, 1616–1622. [CrossRef]
46. Hawke, T.J.; Garry, D.J. Myogenic satellite cells: Physiology to molecular biology. *J. Appl. Physiol.* **2001**, *91*, 534–551. [CrossRef] [PubMed]
47. Barton, E.R. Viral expression of insulin-like growth factor-I isoforms promotes different responses in skeletal muscle. *J. Appl. Physiol.* **2006**, *100*, 1778–1784. [CrossRef] [PubMed]
48. Wernbom, M.; Augustsson, J.; Raastad, T. Ischemic strength training: A low-load alternative to heavy resistance exercise? *Scand. J. Med. Sci. Sports* **2008**, *18*, 401–416. [CrossRef]
49. Abe, T.; Yasuda, T.; Midorikawa, T.; Sato, Y.; Kearns, C.F.; Inoue, K.; Koizumi, K.; Ishii, N. Skeletal muscle size and circulating IGF-1 are increased after two weeks of twice daily "KAATSU" resistance training. *Int. J. KAATSU Train. Res.* **2005**, *1*, 6–12. [CrossRef]
50. West, D.W.; Kujbida, G.W.; Moore, D.R.; Atherton, P.; Burd, N.A.; Padzik, J.P.; De Lisio, M.; Tang, J.E.; Parise, G.; Rennie, M.J.; et al. Resistance exercise-induced increases in putative anabolic hormones do not enhance muscle protein synthesis or intracellular signalling in young men. *J. Physiol.* **2009**, *587*, 5239–5247. [CrossRef]
51. Fujita, S.; Abe, T.; Drummond, M.J.; Cadenas, J.G.; Dreyer, H.C.; Sato, Y.; Volpi, E.; Rasmussen, B.B. Blood flow restriction during lowintensity resistance exercise increases S6K1 phos-phorylation and muscle protein synthesis. *J. Appl. Physiol.* **2007**, *103*, 903–910. [CrossRef]
52. Wernbom, M.; Paulsen, G.; Bjørnsen, T.M.; Cumming, K.; Raastad, T. Risk of muscle damage with blood flow-restricted exercise should not be overlooked. *Clin. J. Sport Med.* **2021**, *31*, 223–224. [CrossRef] [PubMed]
53. Renzi, C.P.; Tanaka, H.; Sugawara, J. Effects of leg blood flow restriction during walking on cardiovascular function. *Med. Sci. Sports Exerc.* **2010**, *42*, 726–732. [CrossRef] [PubMed]
54. Pearson, S.J.; Hussain, S.R. A review on the mechanisms of blood-flow restriction resistance training-induced muscle hyper-trophy. *Sports Med.* **2015**, *45*, 187–200. [CrossRef] [PubMed]
55. Kawada, S.; Ishii, N. Skeletal muscle hypertrophy after chronic restriction of venous blood flow in rats. *Med. Sci. Sports Exerc.* **2005**, *37*, 1144–1150. [CrossRef] [PubMed]
56. Pope, Z.K.; Willardson, J.M.; Schoenfeld, B.J. Exercise and blood flow restriction. *J. Strength Cond. Res.* **2013**, *27*, 2914–2926. [CrossRef]
57. Yasuda, T.; Brechue, W.F.; Fujita, T.; Shirakawa, J.; Sato, Y.; Abe, T. Muscle activation during low-intensity muscle contractions with restricted blood flow. *J. Sports Sci.* **2009**, *27*, 479–489. [CrossRef]
58. Yasuda, T.; Loenneke, J.; Ogasawara, R.; Abe, T. Influence of continuous or intermittent blood flow restriction on muscle activation during low-intensity multiple sets of resistance exercise. *Acta Physiol. Hung.* **2013**, *100*, 419–426. [CrossRef]
59. Laurentino, G.C.; Ugrinowitsch, C.; Roschel, H.; Aoki, M.S.; Soares, A.G.; Neves, M.; Aihara, A.Y.; Fernandes, A.D.R.C.; Tricoli, V. Strength training with blood flow restriction diminishes myostatin gene expression. *Med. Sci. Sports Exerc.* **2012**, *44*, 406–412. [CrossRef]
60. Goldfarb, A.H.; Garten, R.S.; Chee, P.D.M.; Cho, C.; Reeves, G.V.; Hollander, D.B.; Thomas, C.; Aboudehen, K.S.; Francois, M.; Kraemer, R.R. Resistance exercise effects on blood glutathione status and plasma protein carbonyls: Influence of partial vascular occlusion. *Eur. J. Appl. Physiol.* **2008**, *104*, 813–819. [CrossRef]

Disclaimer/Publisher's Note: The statements, opinions and data contained in all publications are solely those of the individual author(s) and contributor(s) and not of MDPI and/or the editor(s). MDPI and/or the editor(s) disclaim responsibility for any injury to people or property resulting from any ideas, methods, instructions or products referred to in the content.

MDPI
St. Alban-Anlage 66
4052 Basel
Switzerland
www.mdpi.com

Journal of Clinical Medicine Editorial Office
E-mail: jcm@mdpi.com
www.mdpi.com/journal/jcm

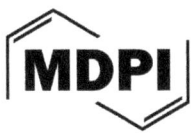

Disclaimer/Publisher's Note: The statements, opinions and data contained in all publications are solely those of the individual author(s) and contributor(s) and not of MDPI and/or the editor(s). MDPI and/or the editor(s) disclaim responsibility for any injury to people or property resulting from any ideas, methods, instructions or products referred to in the content.

www.ingramcontent.com/pod-product-compliance
Lightning Source LLC
LaVergne TN
LVHW070557100526
838202LV00012B/492